FAST
THERAPY

FAST THERAPY

**A 10-DAY SELF-HEALING PROGRAM
FOR MINDBODY CHANGE**

CAMILLA GRIGGERS, PHD

WATERSIDE PUBLISHING
CARDIFF BY THE SEA, CALIFORNIA

Copyright © 2024 by Camilla Griggers

www.camillagriggers.com

All rights reserved. This book or any portion thereof may not be reproduced or used in any manner whatsoever without the express written permission of the publisher except for the use of brief quotations in articles and book reviews.

NO AI TRAINING: Without in any way limiting the author's [and publisher's] exclusive rights under copyright, any use of this publication to "train" generative artificial intelligence (AI) technologies to generate text is expressly prohibited. The author reserves all rights to license uses of this work for generative AI training and development of machine learning language models.

First Printing, 2024

Cover photograph by Kevin Fitzgerald.

ISBN-13: 978-1-962984-18-8

Waterside Productions
2055 Oxford Ave
Cardiff, CA 92007
www.waterside.com

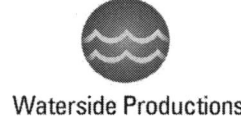

Waterside Productions

DEDICATION

To Gail Shepherd, who taught me to go deeper still to listen beneath the words for the body's truth.

To Rachel Flournoy, who taught me the need to stay in touch and reach out a helping hand to young people who are struggling and need our empathy and care.

To everyone who says they're fine when they're not.

And to all those who know they're not fine and need help fast to turn themselves around.

Contents

DEDICATION	5
PREFAST	11
PART ONE: EMBODIED	15
Chapter 1 GUIDELINES FOR FAST THERAPY	17
Chapter 2 SETTING AN INTENTION TO CHANGE	27
PART TWO: FAST	43
Chapter 3 FAST INSTRUCTIONS	45
PART THREE: THERAPY	77
Chapter 4 MOUTHPEACE — Session One	79
Chapter 5 All EARS — Session Two	95
Chapter 6 EYES WIDE OPEN — Session Three	109
Chapter 7 SKIN DEEP — Session Four	123

Chapter 8 IN TOUCH — Session Five	133
Chapter 9 GUT FEELINGS — Session Six	143
Chapter 10 FACE TO FACE — Session Seven	157
Chapter 11 HEARTFELT — Session Eight	169
Chapter 12 SCAR TISSUE — Session Nine	181
Chapter 13 LANDING ON YOUR FEET — Session Ten	195
AFTERFAST	207
ACKNOWLEDGEMENTS	213
About the Author	216

Fasting is a way to faster healing.
— RUDOLF STEINER

PREFAST

Ten years ago, I went to visit my cousin, Natalie Boss in Greenville, South Carolina, so she could walk me through my first 10-day nutritional wet fast—the one I show you in this book. As a colon hydrotherapist, Natalie knows how important detoxification and elimination of waste are to lifelong health and wellbeing.

"How easy is that?" Natalie said. "Just stop chewing food for 10 days to cleanse your colon and your liver, the Giver of Life." She was talking to me without looking at me as we walked down the street in the morning sunshine headed to her favorite cafe. Both of us were, at that time in our lives, shamelessly addicted to coffee.

She was giving me a pep talk before starting the 10-day liquid nutritional fast—her favorite kind. It nourishes and hydrates your gut with nutrient-rich drinks, eliminates fecal waste from your colon and metabolic waste from your liver, it flushes your kidneys and bladder, and gives your gastrointestinal tract time to heal while burning body fat. It's efficient, effective and safe. In ten days, you lose somewhere between 5 to 10 lbs. of fat and waste depending on how much you have. And just about anyone can do it. Natalie suddenly turned on a dime to face me, making eye contact. *"Drink before you're hungry,"* she said. Then she gave me a knowing look. I realized she was waiting for me to give her a thumbs up or say *"Roger"* to verify I got the memo.

My cousin could be a character out of a Flannery O'Connor story. She's a colon hydrotherapist who likes to quote the Bible who graduated from Georgia Tech as an engineer. In college, she was interested in environmental engineering, however once she learned that basically meant managing sewage, she balked. She laughs about it now, because a healing crisis in her thirties led her to pivot from being an engineer to becoming a colon hydrotherapist. Given her background, it's not surprising that she sees ill health as a personal waste management problem that is connected to our larger environmental waste management problem. Helping people manage their own waste became Natalie's calling.

For her, colon hydrotherapy is a simple human engineering solution to the challenge of too much waste and toxicity. She prays every day that young engineers and industrial designers out there like her niece who graduated from Georgia Tech will integrate health and ecological stewardship into engineering and design solutions to help create a sustainable future we can all live well in.

Natalie and I both made the pivot into wellness practices the same way. We fell ill and realized we had to do something to heal ourselves and prevent becoming seriously ill again. Somewhere along the way, the healing journey turns into a healing practice, especially when you realize the extent to which your healing crisis—in our cases from reproductive tumors that left us both infertile—is the same healing crisis affecting millions and millions of other women. Some of us are naturally called to help. And some of us are willing to touch the problem in the flesh.

My cousin has beautiful long blonde hair, and she's fit because she's always moving. She's an advanced yogi and a daunting ballroom dancer. And she swims laps like a fish. She also fasts for 10 days once or twice a year, whenever she feels the need. So she burns lean. When she walks by you can't help but notice her; she has a sensual swagger that looks like she's practicing a dance move in her head.

When it comes to fasting, Natalie is always willing to join in the adventure. And it is always an adventure, because you don't know exactly what is going to come up—except that you do sort of know, because, after all, it's your *shit*. Still, it can take you by surprise, especially in a culture where people are used to flushing their toxic waste down the toilet without looking at it, assuming it will just magically disappear no matter how foul.

The emergence of Fast Therapy

As a somatic therapist, specializing in somatic-emotional release work, it didn't take many times fasting to realize the potential for doing therapeutic work during a fast. Fasting creates a state of consciousness where the veil is lifted for a short time on your psychological attachments to habitual behaviors that can side-track your self-care skills and send you down the path toward chronic bodymind ill health. Relief is often the first emotion that comes up, and with each day that goes by on a fast, hope for healthy change in your life wells up from within you.

After a few days of freedom from consuming and digesting, your head clears. It feels like you've lifted the lid off your mind as your attention shifts from busy thoughts (many of them the same thoughts you had yesterday) to what you are feeling in your body in the present moment. It feels like lifting the lid off blocked emotions too, letting them release so that your feelings can flow and express freely again. So many of us need that because we live in a culture where people typically suppress their emotions, holding them in, hiding them or swallowing them down with a coffee, drink or comfort food, or displacing them onto something they feel they can control like a cigarette, a joint, or a drug that can end up seducing one toward addiction.

When you fast for 10 days and break these habitual attachments, you trigger a state of detoxification and renewal that is mental, physical, emotional and spiritual all at the same time. For this reason, it's common during fasting to experience somatic-emotional releases that permanently shift your thinking, feelings and behaviors. In just 10 days, you change from within, sometimes quite dramatically.

One day in a natural evolution, I began offering nutritional wet fasting instructions to my clients who came to me with chronic physical and psychic pain, and we would do bodymind integration exercises and hands-on somatic-emotional release sessions before, during and after the 10-day nutritional fast. In that work we did together, Fast Therapy was born. In this book, I share this body psychology approach to self-healing, showing you how to be your own somatic therapist to do Fast Therapy at home.

PART 1
EMBODIED

Chapter 1

GUIDELINES FOR FAST THERAPY

On being triggered

"Triggered" is a word that is often used pejoratively to mean acting irritated and agitated when something triggers a somatic-emotional memory of a past trauma in which you act out bits and pieces of the original trauma in the present moment. However, the word also has a positive meaning when something triggers a healing crisis that ends well or stimulates a response in the present moment that is healthy and adaptive. If you get triggered doing any of these exercises, it's not the end of the world. In fact, it may be the beginning of a healing crisis in which you have an opportunity to heal something deep inside you that needs more love and care.

Suppressing your emotions can make you sick

We all know emotions can come up during bodywork. You can imagine what happens when you take 10 days to cleanse your visceral organs of the waste of the past. *Crap moves, comes to the surface, and gets purged.* Suppressed emotions from embodied memories—some of them traumatic—are laden with the impulse to discharge. Let them. There's an emotional detox that accompanies physical detox. If you've learned to bottle up your emotions, sit on them, swallow them down, hide them, manage them or in any way suppress them, understand that emotions are energy, and energy never just disappears, it ***moves***. So emotional energy will come up and express even if you try to suppress it. When feelings rise up, surrender to them, let them express and release. Trust me, it's healthier to get them off your chest, off your back, and out the door.

Ethics of caretaking

When you reach out with the intention to help during some of the Fast Therapy partner exercises — or as you practice and apply the exercises with people in your life — it's important to have an ethics of care in place to prevent hindering when you thought you were helping. I like to refer to a favorite quote by Ram Dass for guidance. In it, he uses an example of handing a glass of water to someone in need.

> *"Let's say I give water to a sick person. I hand them a glass of water. How many levels can I hand them a glass of water from? Where is my heart in handing them a glass of water? Where is my identity in the glass of water? Who am I handing the glass of water to? Who am I in the situation? Where is God in that? How is emptiness related in the form? That's all inherent in the way the water is handed from one person to another. So in a way, saying the service is in handing the glass of water is only part of what the service is. Service exists in the nature of the interaction so that the interaction between two human beings frees everybody."*

Remember these words of wisdom whenever you reach out with a green juice or cup of hot detox tea to help someone in need. What is most important is that the interaction between both people is liberating. Everybody is freed by it. It takes practice. Be willing to practice. When you receive kindness and empathy, it is easier to trust. When you give kindness and empathy, it is easier to be trusted.

This principle applies to any traumatized, wounded or ill part of yourself that you've been hiding away that may be listening right now.

Preventive self-care

Once you recognize and accept the bodymind connection for what it is, you understand why, when spiritual teachers tell us to hold our anger like a baby, they really mean cradle our liver like a baby, feed it, and clean its waste. This adage applies to all our visceral organs, because each organ regulates specific emotions as part of how it functions. When you feel out of balance emotionally and mentally and suffer physical pain and discomfort, listen to the organ crying out for attention to discern what you need to come to back to balance again. If you feel depressed, cradle your colon like a baby, nourish it and clean its waste. If you feel chronically anxious and stressed, cradle your kidneys like a baby and take care of them.

Most importantly, if you've fallen out of balance or even fallen ill in some part of yourself, forgive yourself now for not paying attention before, for forgetting to take care of yourself, or being unable to find the resources to help yourself or someone you love. It doesn't matter that you missed opportunities in the past to take action to improve the situation. What matters is what you do now in the present.

What if you're working with a talk therapist while doing Fast Therapy?

If you work with a talk therapist and you're thinking *"oh, but my therapist isn't a body-centered psychotherapist or a somatic therapist,"* look for one and you'll find one. They're everywhere. But you don't have to. If you want support while you're doing Fast Therapy, schedule time with your therapist while you're fasting and bring all the sensations and feelings that come up for you into your therapist's office. Take the lead yourself in your talk therapy sessions to bring your body more into the conversation. I guarantee you you'll have a deep session with a lot of insights and emotional movement.

As long as you verbalize what you're feeling in your sensory and emotional body, your talk therapist will be able to follow along wherever you go. And good therapists understand body language, whether they are trained in body-centered approaches or not. Touch your own embodiment, laying a listening hand on where you feel tension, pain and discomfort, ask that part of you what it would say if it had words, and then listen with curious ears and an open mind and heart. You'll have plenty to talk about with your talk therapist that keeps your body directly engaged in the conversation.

Seeing, feeling and touching the bodymind connections

Look at the 4 images below. Scan each one in its entirety. Next, read each word on the page mindfully while touching the word with the index finger of one hand and placing the other hand on the part of your body the words refer to (kidneys are on the back side of you.) Open your mind and heart to see and feel the bodymind connections. Maybe some you're aware of, maybe some are new to you. Have fun connecting the dots between body, mind and emotions.

After you've spent some time with all 4 images, answer the 3 questions at the end of this chapter.

MESSENGER HORMONES

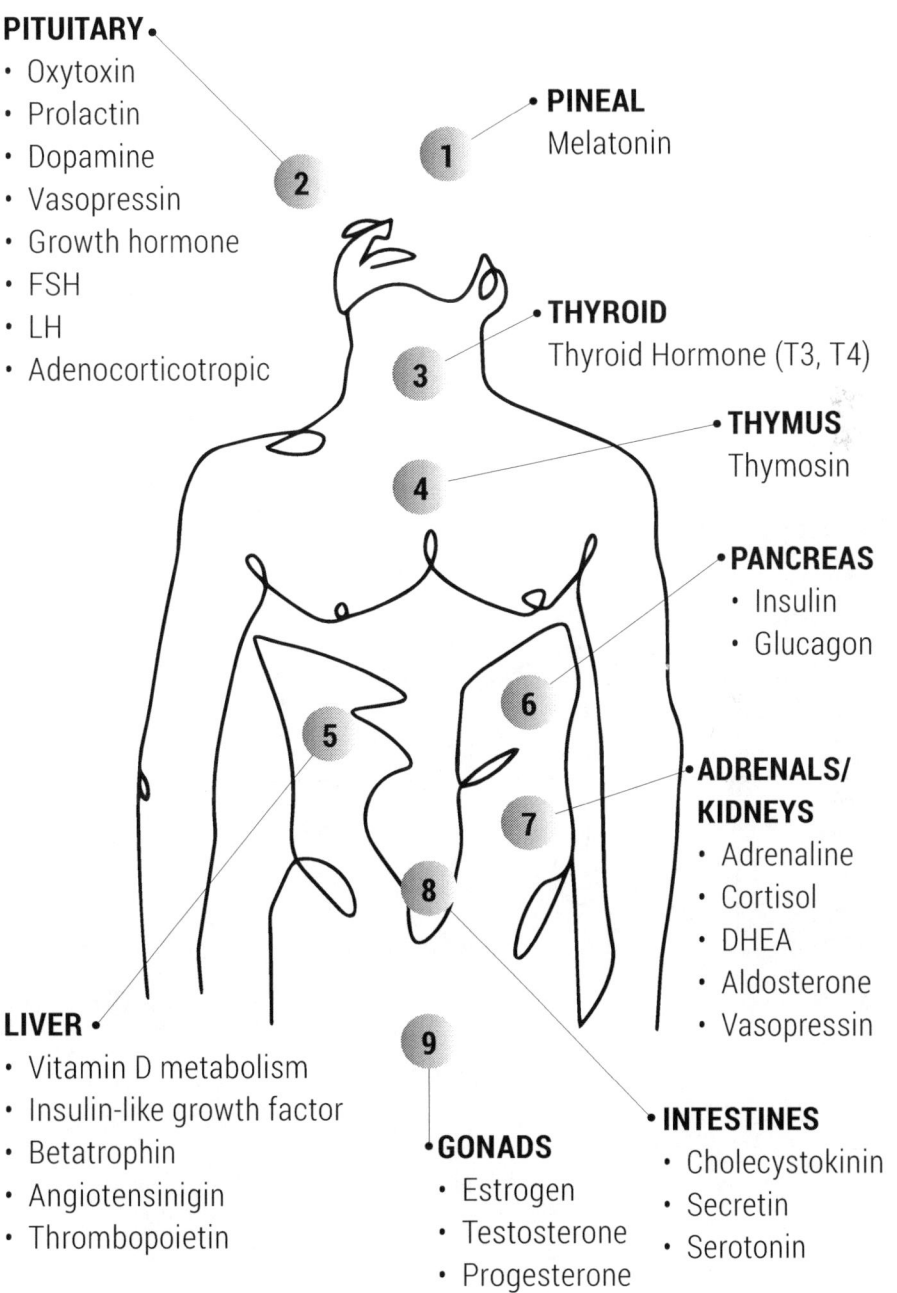

PITUITARY
- Oxytoxin
- Prolactin
- Dopamine
- Vasopressin
- Growth hormone
- FSH
- LH
- Adenocorticotropic

PINEAL
Melatonin

THYROID
Thyroid Hormone (T3, T4)

THYMUS
Thymosin

PANCREAS
- Insulin
- Glucagon

ADRENALS/ KIDNEYS
- Adrenaline
- Cortisol
- DHEA
- Aldosterone
- Vasopressin

LIVER
- Vitamin D metabolism
- Insulin-like growth factor
- Betatrophin
- Angiotensinigin
- Thrombopoietin

GONADS
- Estrogen
- Testosterone
- Progesterone

INTESTINES
- Cholecystokinin
- Secretin
- Serotonin

UNSTRESSED EMOTIONS

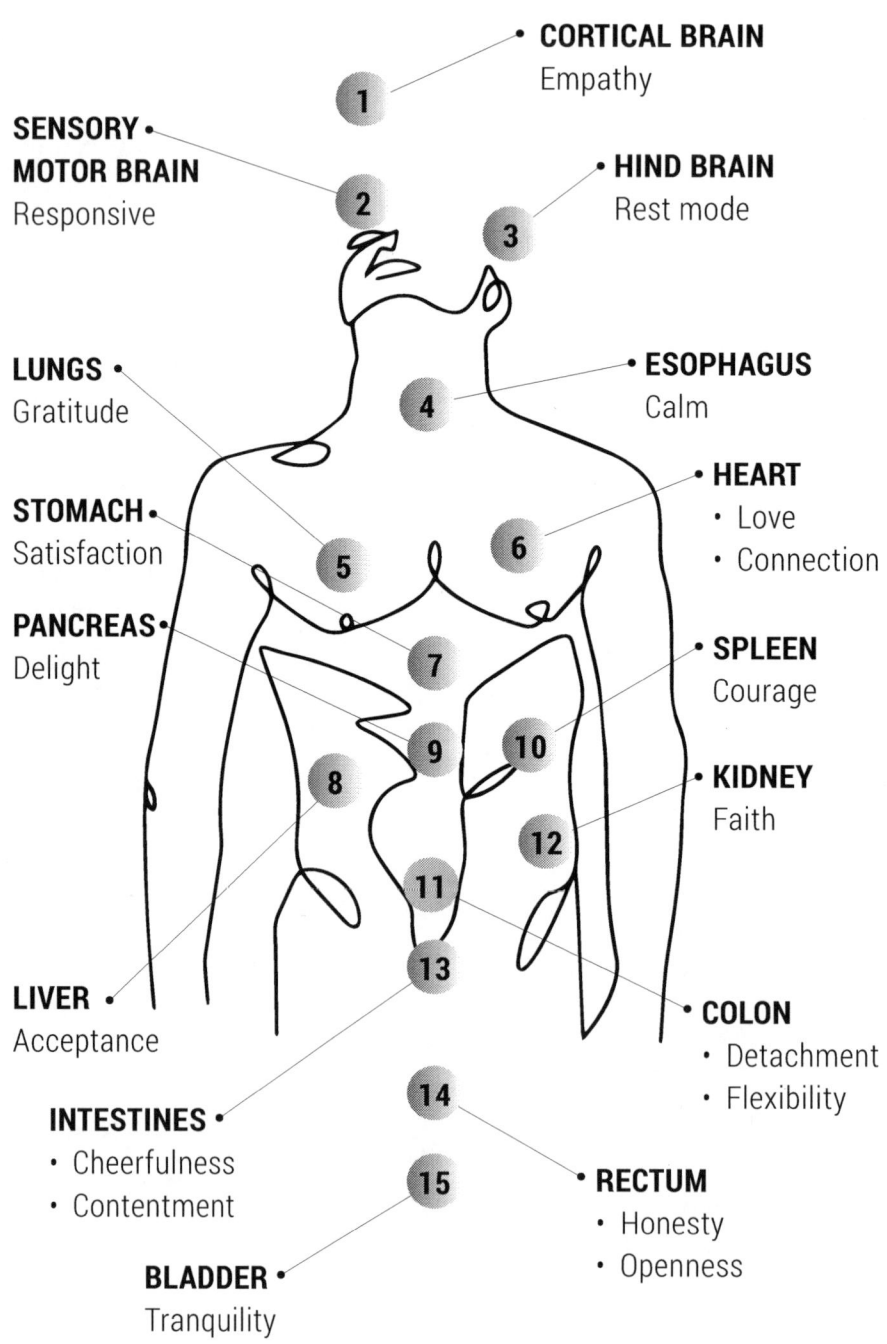

STRESSED EMOTIONS

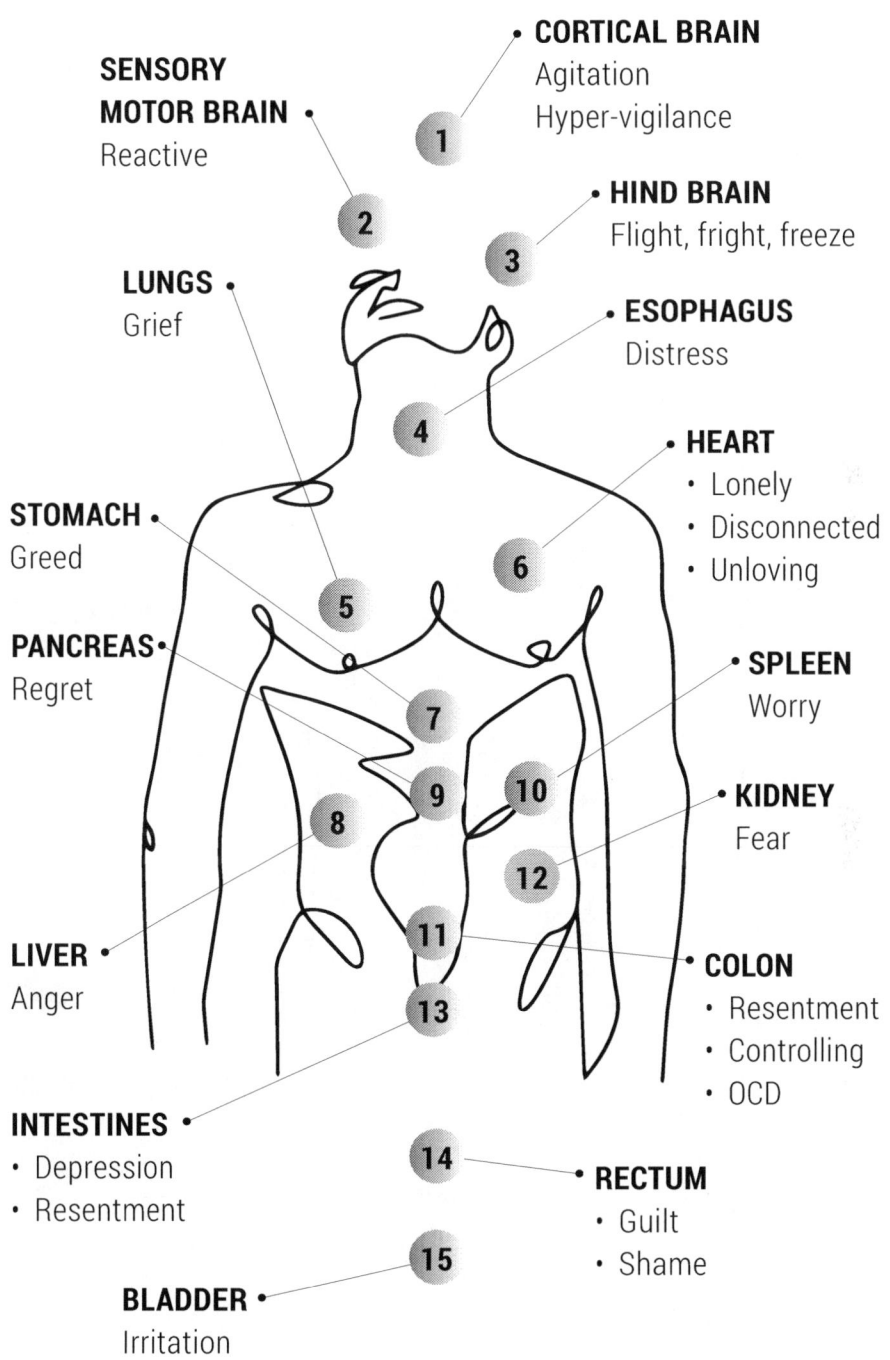

IMMUNE SYSTEM

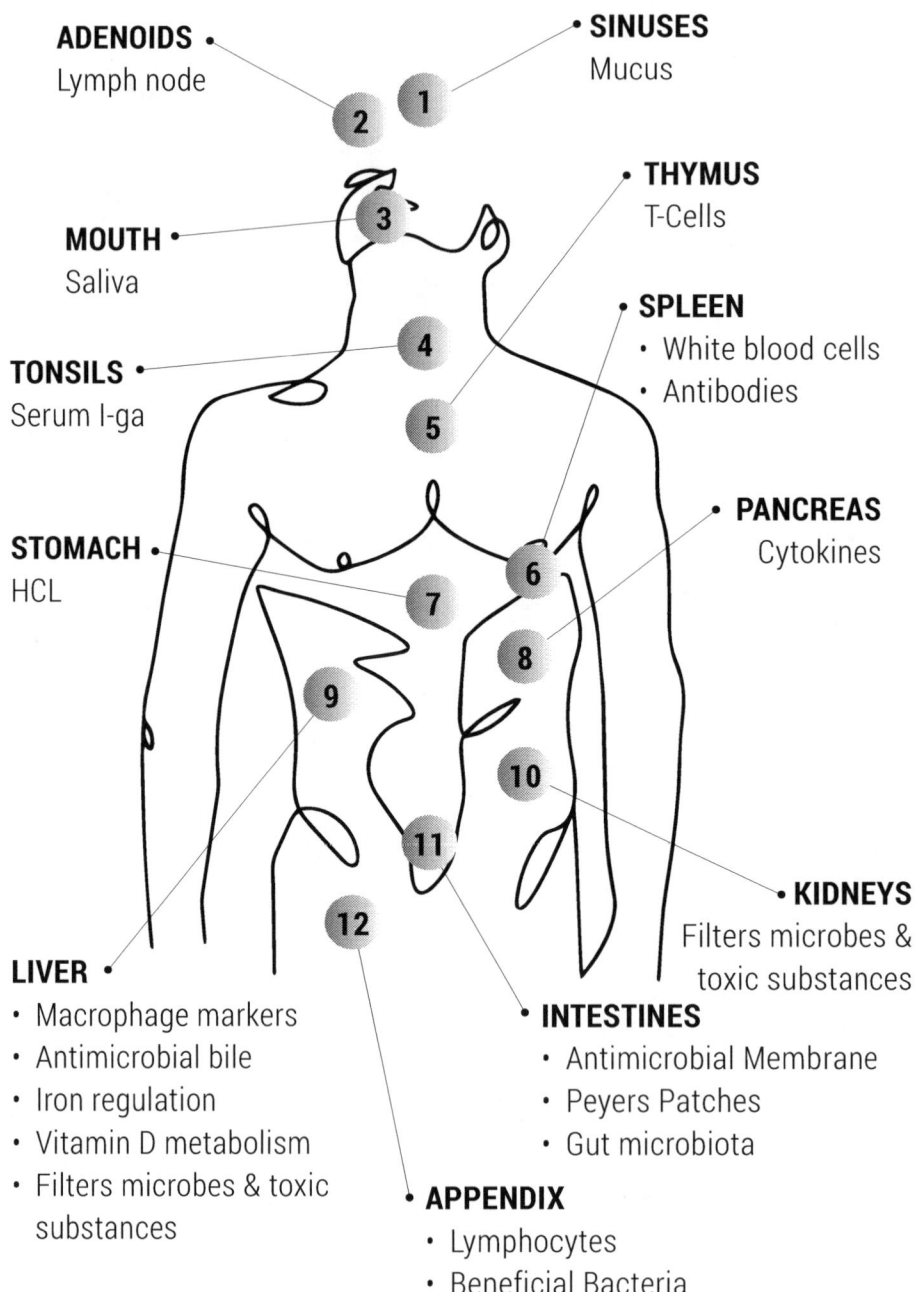

Exercise: Identify parts of yourself in need of more attention and care

Identify a chronically blocked and stressed emotion you want to release during Fast Therapy.

Blocked emotion:

_____

_____

Identify a chronically stressed organ or gland you would like to take care of during Fast Therapy.

Stressed organ or gland:

_____

_____

Identify a habitual illness-causing thought pattern you would like to change during Fast Therapy.

Habitual thought pattern:

_____

_____

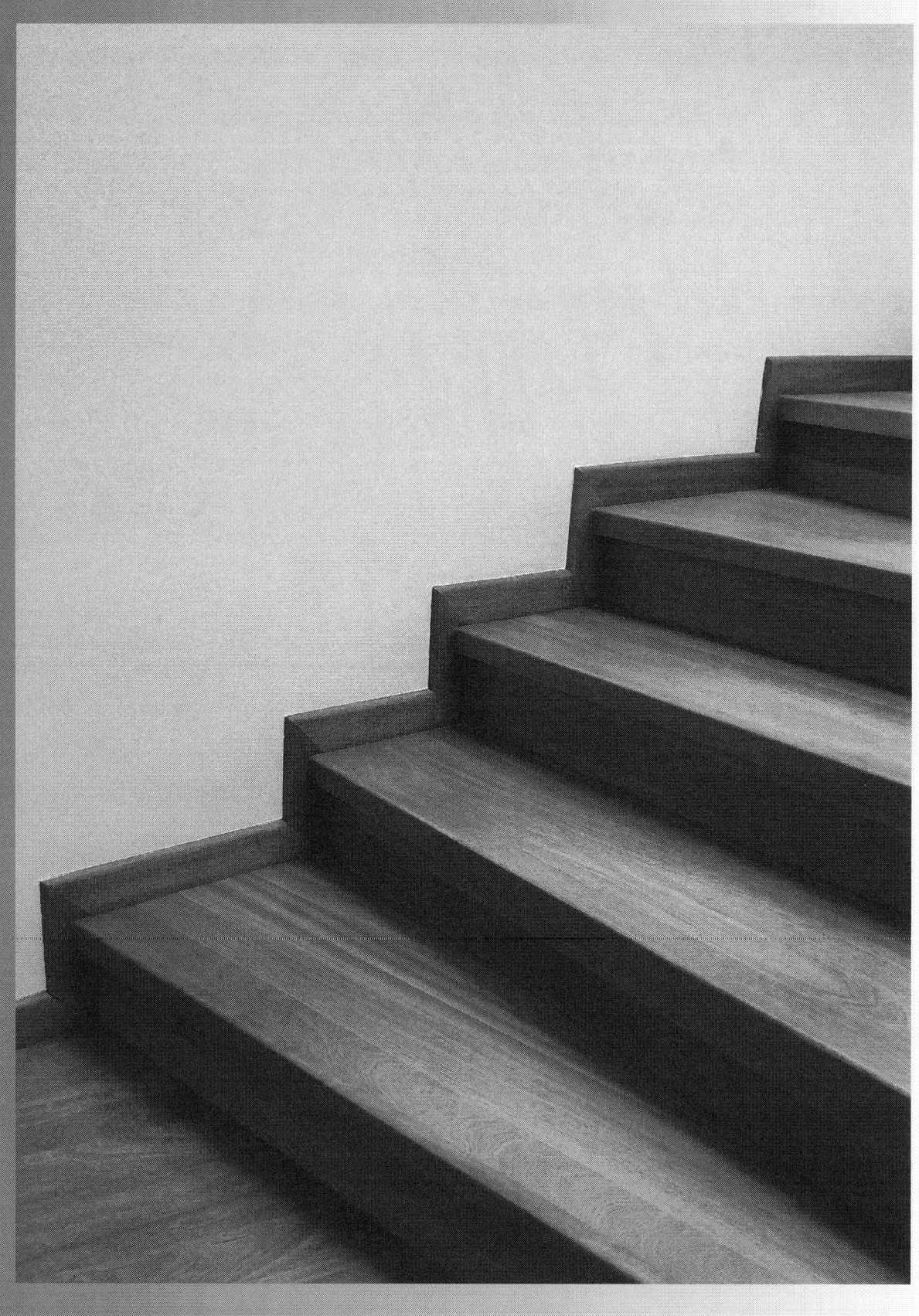

Chapter 2

SETTING AN INTENTION TO CHANGE

Before you start anything important in your life, it helps to set a clear intention. By visualizing what you want to achieve, you can leverage the bodymind connection to optimize your results. For most Westerners, because of our postmodern condition in which the mind/body split has been institutionalized throughout society, we tend to think about setting an intention as something we do mentally. But in somatic therapy where our guiding principle is the bodymind connection, we know the intention we want to set isn't just in our mind. It's in our body.

Setting a somatic intention

F. M. Alexander, creator of the Alexander Technique in the 1890s and a founding father of somatic therapies, used the example of climbing stairs to explain how we set an intention in our body. The lesson became a classic teaching in somatic education and has been put to good use by somatic therapists, coaches, actors, dancers, musicians and professional athletes. It can be used by anyone who wants to optimize their performance doing anything, and we can use it to optimize our performance doing 10 days of fasting therapy.

When we climb a set of stairs in our life, what are we doing exactly? Well, we know what we aren't doing. We aren't rushing over and throwing ourselves at the bottom stair, focusing all our attention there so that when we look up, we feel unprepared for all the stairs still left to climb. Nor are we fixing our gaze at the top of the stairs to the point that we don't see the bottom stair, and trip on the bottom stair in our eagerness to reach the top. Whatever we do, we know we want to keep our balance throughout the climb to prevent falling down the stairs and hurting ourselves. I think all of us know that if we overthink it, we only make it more difficult to get to the top of whatever stairs we're trying to climb. While none of us ever wants to fall down, worrying about falling down, focusing on falling down, and anxiously fearing falling down all increase the chances of making a misstep and falling down the stairs.

Watch out what you envision, right?

Face it. If you feel fear when you go to climb stairs in your life, you'll have to face that fear to get up your stairs. It helps to acknowledge that the risk of falling down is real. We all have a primal fear of falling down for good reason. We are wise to take the risk seriously. I'll be the first to admit, it takes courage to climb some of the stairs facing us these days, when more than 50% of Americans already have one or more chronic illnesses, including mental illnesses. If you're paying attention to the stats, you know the odds are turning against all of us.

To keep you from sitting frozen in fear and doing nothing when doing nothing is how we got in our current healthcare crisis, the embodied therapy sessions in Part Three of this book nudge you to get up and move through the emotions, sensations and blockages you might experience day by day as you fast. I guide you to do some bodymind integration to embody positive changes faster. Trust that once you start your Fast Therapy, you're going to get a lot of support every day once you get into the fast. But first, you need to get yourself ready to actually fast, meaning jump in, or step in, or wade in...however you need and want to do it to *get in your fast*. Sometimes it takes guts over fear. Sometimes it takes faith. But most of all, you need to believe you can do it.

For those of you who tend to have fretful negative thoughts just when it comes time to dream big and take action, I want to encourage you to envision your Fast Therapy experience in the most positive and healing way you can. I promise you will get more and more relief from obsessive negative thinking as you move from Day 1 to Day 10 of your fast, because, as you're going to learn firsthand, that kind of anxious compulsive fretting has everything to do with how constipated and congested your colon is, how stressed your kidneys are, and how out of balance your gut microbiome is, since most of the neurohormone transmitters used by our brain are made in our gut.

I assure you by the end of 10 days of fasting therapy, your colon and liver will be empty and clean, your mind and your gut will be clear and calm, and your heart will feel open and connected. I can tell you all that. But if you've never fasted before, you have to get all the way to the top of the stairs yourself to experience what I'm describing.

So what exactly *are* we doing when we climb stairs in our life to reach a goal?

F. M. Alexander's big insight that is used today by world-class athletes and performers around the world was that most of the work is done before you ever start your climb. From the moment you enter a space and lay your eyes on the stairs, you imagine yourself enacting the sequence of actions required to reach the top and organize your parts to do what you have already envisioned. You visually scan the stairs from bottom to top and back down and then focus your gaze on the horizon and zoom out, mapping your body into that space. When you visualize what you're doing in this way, it feels less like looking at a 2D Instagram selfie and more like being inside of a 3D hologram.

Gravity and momentum

Let's go back to our Alexander Technique lesson. What we humans lose in stability by standing up vertically on two legs we gain in agility. Because we stand up tall, we have the ability to see what's coming early, move quickly in any direction, and change direction on a dime. We can't outrun a tiger, but we can out-maneuver it. Because of our vertical posture, we can create a lot of momentum extremely fast by moving our head in the direction we want to go, including upward momentum to climb a tree if we need to. With momentum, we can bend gravity. Without momentum, gravity bends us.

Okay, what's the takeaway? If you want to climb some personal stairs right now in your life, whatever that means for you, you'll need momentum. And I tell you from first-hand experience, Fast Therapy is a way to create a lot of momentum fast.

Bringing mind, body and emotions into sync

F. M. Alexander's "*Aha*" moment came during his own healing crisis as a young stage actor who suffered from chronic laryngitis. His famous method for somatic therapy came to him when he realized his mental map of what he was doing was different from what he was physically doing in his body when he was on stage. That incongruency between what he thought he was doing and what he actually was doing with his body was causing him to go on stage to climb his stairs and repeatedly fall down the stairs in front of his audience. His voice would go hoarse, and he would eventually lose it. It was the opposite of what he wanted.

At first, F. M. Alexander thought there was something wrong with his vocal cords and that he had a physical problem. But treating his physical problem got him nowhere. Eventually he realized that his problem was certainly physical, but it was also in his mind. He realized he mistakenly thought he needed to stretch his neck forward to project his voice on stage, and so he put unnecessary physical stress on his vocal cords. As soon as he stopped doing that unnatural forward motion with his head, his vocal cords were fine, and he could project his voice on stage without strain.

At this point, F. M. Alexander decided to leave behind his acting career to become a pioneer in the field of somatic therapy. He had found his remedy. The Alexander Technique for which he became famous is a method for developing somatic awareness and changing somatic patterns by creating a feedback loop to help your mind get integrated with your body. It's a body-first approach to education and therapy that's the opposite of mind over matter. Instead, mind and body are brought into sync.

Luckily, we all intuitively know how to stand up and climb a set of stairs if we are able bodied. Children figure it out quickly as they develop enough coordination and balance. Even if you have an injury of some kind that requires physical therapy to go up and down stairs, the physical therapist is simply helping your body remember what you already know how to do. If you developed compensations along the way to cope with injuries, traumas or illnesses that now are blocking you from full function when you set about to climb stairs in your life, a physical therapist or somatic therapist can help you release those compensations from your body memory to recover your natural function again, and even better, to optimize your performance.

The same is true of fasting. You don't really need to learn how to fast, even if you've never done a fast before, because we all know how to fast if we've ever had a fever and intuitively stopped eating. We lie down in bed, let all our energy go to our immune system to fight off an infection, and surrender to the fact that it's time to heal, not eat. We respect the natural wisdom of that process and get out of our own way to help our body do what it knows how to do.

In the same way, we all know how to fast when we don't have any food or we're running out of food. Our body knows instinctively what to do to get through the experience. We naturally turn inward to conserve energy and water and become introspective while we get hyper-focused on sourcing the essentials we need to survive. Our body's innate understanding of fasting also explains why we naturally don't want to eat a big meal before we go on stage for a life-changing event where we want to perform at our best. Sitting down to enjoy a fine meal happens *after* the performance of a lifetime.

By the way, bringing awareness to a dysfunctional sequence so that you can make a healthy adjustment to your sequencing can be a liberating way to somatically repattern habitual behaviors that have become maladaptive. If you know you have a habitual pattern that is dysfunctional and has caused physical, emotional and psychic pain in your life, identify that somatic pattern you want to repattern here. Maybe it's something like, when I get sad, I eat comfort food, or I drink another glass of wine (alcohol is a depressant). Or whatever it is. Maybe when you get anxious or bored, you smoke a cigarette, or snort a drug up your nose or pop a pill. Or maybe you just sit too much or talk too much and so forget to exercise, or you forget to eat when you're hungry until you're "hangry."

Whatever it is, identify it here.

My habitual pattern I need to repattern for better bodymind health and happiness:

_____

_____

Climbing styles will vary based on situation and motivation

Why you want to get to the top of your stairs doesn't really matter. One person who did Fast Therapy was motivated to finally do something about his high blood pressure that had him and everyone around him worried sick. Another wanted relief from embarrassing intestinal gas that made going out on a dinner date an ordeal instead of a pleasure. Still another wanted to let go of drinking alcohol every night. Another who is an actress wanted to look and feel her best before ending a series she'd starred in for years while starting a new film.

Everyone has a different motivation to do Fast Therapy. One person walked away after 10 days of fasting minus the 10 pounds of extra weight she was tired of carrying around, along with chronic constipation. For another, it was leaving behind 20 pounds of habitual over-eating. Another person was in a career pivot seeking an inward journey to find spiritual guidance about her higher purpose in life — and why she was still single. Others were seeking relief from chronic pain, or were responding to an early warning from a lab report or from their physician. One client wanted to get to the bottom of chronic bladder infections that blocked her from a happy sex life and had her on rounds and rounds of antibiotics that left her irritated, controlling, depressed and anxious, but never completely healed her poor bladder of irritation and inflammation. Another client wanted to get rid of a chronic stabbing pain in his back along with a memory of betrayal that kept him single when he didn't really want to be single anymore.

There are so many different reasons to want to do a bodymind reset with Fast Therapy. Whatever it is, own your intention and commit to it. Maybe you're a fitness buff, athlete or biohacker in pursuit of optimal bodymind performance. Maybe you want to turn around an illness that is becoming chronic or prevent a chronic disease in your family history. For some it's healing from addiction. The point is, every body is different. Every body's story is different. The stairs and the climb will be different for everyone. For some it may feel easy, and they may breeze through 10 days of fasting therapy feeling fantastic. For others, it may be a struggle from Day 1. Remember, just taking the journey for 10 days to give yourself time to cleanse and restore is your ultimate destination. If you do Fast Therapy for 10 days, *you will change*. It's guaranteed because for starters, you'll liberate yourself from walking around stewing in your own crap.

Naturally, the way you approach your fast is going to be very personal. If you're recovering from an injury or illness, for example, you might take it one step at a time, slow and steady, with one hand holding onto the handrail. If you're an athlete, fitness buff or biohacker, you might glide through the fast in record time hands-free, with minimal expenditure of energy and perfect technique. And if rushing flood waters are threatening to wash you downstream, you might see yourself scrambling into the fast pell-mell using whatever energy you can muster to dive into the experience.

However, if you are a bride getting ready to climb the stairs into a sacred sanctuary where you will marry your beloved in front of your family and friends, you might imagine climbing the stairs of Fast Therapy slowly with grace and composure, carefully trailing the train of a wedding gown behind you. Or maybe you are in search of a rite of passage for personal transformation to grow a part of yourself up, or to find your way through an emotional or spiritual healing crisis. Whatever challenge you face in life, visualize yourself having already reached your goal on Day 10 of your Fast Therapy.

Fasting with others

If you feel you need support, ask a friend or family member to do Fast Therapy with you. If you see someone who looks like they need support, ask them if they want to join you for a healing journey. It's always an enlightening adventure to do Fast Therapy as a couple or a group, I assure you of that. And it's easier to manage the daily routine if people are sharing the labor of sourcing and prepping the daily drinks. However, be prepared to go forward alone if they decline. If you find yourself waiting for others to start your own self-care, you are dancing with codependency. Fast Therapy is a fast remedy for codependency, because only you control what you put in your mouth and when. And only you can choose to stop eating for 10 days and start drinking nutrient-rich drinks to wash out your waste, nutrient saturate your cells, and restore better health. By taking the lead and instigating change, many people discover that those around them often follow their lead when they are willing to go first.

Fast success stories

For those of you who haven't fasted before, you will find inspiration in some of these testimonials of people who did Fast Therapy and experienced positive, even life-changing results. Their accounts will help you set your intention and envision climbing your stairs before you read the fasting instructions in the next chapter.

"I did the 10-day Fast Therapy challenge twice, and by the second time my results were dramatic. Not only did I lose the 20 lbs. of weight I wanted to lose, but my energy shot up and so did my zest for life. I felt emotionally renewed. For me, it was an experience of personal transformation. I seriously feel like and look like a new person."

"I was so very happy with the results of my first 10-day fast — including kicking a two-year sleeping pill addiction — when the opportunity to do it again arose, I knew it was time for a follow up. The second round of fasting therapy was even better, because I saw the cleansing effects on day 5 all the way past day 10 to day 14. This time long rubbery slime came out. I was delightfully grossed out! My benefits included mental clarity, better sleep & digestion, 9 lbs. of weight loss, emotional balance and peace, not to mention more energy and clearer skin."

"Doing Fast Therapy taught me how to detox my colon, liver and gallbladder. And guess what? The chronic pain in my right shoulder blade went away. Now I know that pain in the back of my shoulder was my dirty gallbladder and liver talking to me. I realized I was walking around for years dehydrated and constipated. When I was guided to do emotional healing work at the same time, I realized I also needed to change how I was in my relationships. Like why I wasn't in one. That really opened my heart and mind."

"Fast therapy completely shifted my relationship to food, my body, and my awareness of self. I realized after 10 days of fasting that I'd been constantly consuming and not really pausing to give myself permission and time to let go. I realized I was addicted to food, to consumption itself. I now honor the process of consuming only what I really need in my core Self and then releasing waste and negative feelings."

"As difficult as fasting was—and I have to be honest, I struggled — I really appreciated the results of it. I'm so glad my sister came to help me. I couldn't have done it without her. For me, the experience of the 10-day fast was transformational. I've been dealing with high blood pressure for years, and recently it had gotten worse to the point that I was seriously worried about myself. Worried I might not see my kids graduate from college. By day 10, I had lost 7 lbs. and my blood pressure reading was 116/70. That's optimal! But more than just physical, fasting was transformative psychologically. There's a merit to austerity, and to making yourself a better person, honoring your Self enough to make healthy changes. That feeling of austerity was something that stayed with me after the fast was over. Now I realize how little I need to be healthy and happy. And my kids were fascinated with all the drinks and everything I was doing while fasting. It felt good showing them I could take care of myself."

These testimonies give you a sense of what it's like after you get to the end of Fast Therapy. In just 10 days, you change your bodymind health for the better. That's fast! That kind of healthy internal change is easily within reach, but only you can do it. It starts when you stop consuming—long enough to clean out your own waste and deal with your own physical and emotional pain. Change doesn't happen in the past. And it doesn't happen in an indefinite future that may never arrive. It happens in the present moment once you start a healing journey by taking action.

A story of family healing

I want to share with you the inspiring story of the sister referenced in the testimonial above, who came to help her brother with his fast. Her brother wasn't the only person in her family that she assisted.

Just as the two-year anniversary of her beloved sister's sudden and rapid demise to brain cancer approached, this inspiring woman did 10-days of Fast Therapy with her husband. Afterwards, she guided her daughter and a dear friend through all 10 days of the fast, and then a few weeks later flew to be with her brother to help him do Fast Therapy. Her husband raced through the experience like the fitness-buff biohacker addicted to adrenaline that he is while learning to let go of being motivated by stress. Her daughter and friend dragged their feet along the way to losing extra pounds of weight and sludge and finding some clarity of mind. And her brother struggled outright physically, emotionally and spiritually with big changes in his life. However, all of them made it through all 10 days and reaped tangible benefits they could see and feel.

This remarkable woman's actions speak louder than words. Obviously, she was moved to take care of the people she loves in a way she couldn't for her sister, because she didn't see her sister's cancer coming. Now she took the lead herself with people in her life. What she did is so important. We can't help the people we love for long if we can't help ourselves first. When she was willing to go first and show the way, she discovered that people in her life chose to follow her lead.

Finding your medicine

There's an ancient story in the oral tradition of the Mohawk Iroquois tribe describing a fast used for a rite of passage, and I want to share it with you now to give you inspiration and guidance as you set your personal intention to do 10 days of fasting therapy. This instructional tale was written down by Aren Akweks and archived in the Six Nations Museum in Onchiota, New York, and later recounted by Allan Macfarian in *Native American Tales and Legends*. But the story has been around for thousands of years.

Since ancient times, it was the practice of the Iroquois tribe that when a boy reached the age of 14 winters, his father would take him to a sacred place in the mountains and leave him for four or five days alone to fast and seek a vision in which the clan's spirit animal, in this case a bear, would visit him in a dream. This vision would provide a clue that would lead the boy to find his personal guardian, something that would be a helper to him for the rest of his life.

During the four or five days of his fast, the boy could drink water to quench his thirst, but he was not allowed to eat any food. After he had completed his fast, seen his vision and found his guardian, the boy would become a man in his own eyes and in the eyes of his tribe. However, there would be no second chance. He would have to complete the fast, have a vision, and find a guardian. The guardian was also referred to as a medicine.

Every day the father would check on his son to see if the spirit of their clan had visited him in a dream and shown him his medicine. When he had found his medicine, the father would escort his son home to their tribe as an adult and no longer a child.

On the morning of the fifth day of the fast, the father of a boy named Otjiera came to check on his son. The boy had craftily built a lodge of young saplings in a balsam forest, covering it with balsam branches to shelter him from the rain. However, his vision had not appeared to him. Otjiera was afraid he would have to return to his village without a guide, so he asked his father in a weak voice for one more day.

That night, a ferocious thunderstorm rolled down the mountain valley in a fierce wind. Sheltering in his lodge in a waking dream state that fasting triggers, Otjiera gathered his courage and faced the storm, asking the thunder to show him his medicine. In an instant, a blinding flash of lightning revealed a large bear standing next to him. Facing his fear and overcoming the impulse to run, he turned around to face the bear. The bear spoke to him, telling him he would receive a medicine on this night that would help not only him, but all his clan.

The boy woke from his vision to hear a horrible screeching sound outside his lodge like nothing he had ever heard before. It sounded monstrous. Facing his fear, he ventured outside to see with his own eyes what could make such a terrifying noise. The howling fierce wind rushing down the mountain was bending two balsam trees together, causing their branches to rub violently against each other. As the boy watched, two branches began to smoke and burst into flames. The sight of fire sent a bolt of fear through him like nothing he had experienced before.

Remembering what his spirit animal had said to him in his vision, Otjiera realized this was the guardian he had asked for. In a flash of insight, he took two small branches of balsam from the ground and rubbed them together violently until a thin trail of smoke rose up, followed by tiny sparks. By using some dry cedar bark and grass, he soon made a fire of his own.

The boy had found his medicine. The story is called "The Discovery of Fire" and tells how fire came to the Mohawk people long ago.

The lesson in this ancient story about fasting still guides us today. Trust there will be challenges and revelations along the way. You may see things you've never seen before. There may be moments when you want to run away in fear. Face your fears. Set an intention for yourself to go away to your sacred mountain (even if that's just your bedroom when other people in your house are eating dinner), build a sacred lodge (be creative), and fast. Ask to be shown your medicine. Take heart knowing that the natural remedy you discover on your journey may help not only you but also your family, friends and even future generations.

Exercise: Identify your challenge

Before you move on to the fasting instructions in the next chapter, it's time to set an intention for yourself. Take a few minutes to identify the stairs facing you that you need to climb.

Write down your personal motivation here. Say what you want.

My motivation:

_____

_____

Once you've identified your motivation, identify what is challenging or blocking you here.

My challenge/blockage:

_____

_____

Now close your eyes and practice silent nasal breathing until you drop down into a meditative state. When you've dropped down into a waking dream state, visualize yourself having already reached the top of your stairs. Remember to visualize a three-dimensional scenario you are in the middle of, doing something you love and feeling great doing it. When you have a clear vision, go to the next chapter to learn how to do a 10-day nutritional wet fast—your medicine.

After your meditative visualization, write your vision down so you can refer to it later.

My vision:

_____

_____

PART 2
FAST

Chapter 3

FAST INSTRUCTIONS

The nutritional wet fast

Nutritional wet fasting is easier than a juice fast (no food just raw vegetable juices), easier than a water fast (no food just water), and easier than a dry fast (no food and no water). I've done all these types of fasts, and they were all useful in different situations for different needs. The easiest and safest of these fasts, especially if this is your first time fasting, is the nutritional wet fast that we cover in this chapter, because you drink a full range of bioavailable essential nutrients every day, which means you are nutrient saturating while detoxing. It's impossible to get truly hungry on a nutritional wet fast.

Not so fast if you're pregnant

Fasting of any kind is not recommended for pregnant women because they need to feed themselves and their baby. Pregnancy is a time to eat the best organic and pasture-grazed whole foods that you can source. It's a time to listen to your gut instinct about what you want and need to consume nutritionally while eliminating nutrient-depleted foods that are inflammatory and constipating.

Fasting *before* conception is good prevention

Whereas fasting during pregnancy is not recommended at all, fasting one or two years *before* conception is the *best* preventive care for both mother and child. Detoxifying and eliminating toxic substances from your body *before* conception is just good prevention, because heavy metals, pesticides, herbicides, petrochemicals and plastics can pass through the placenta, umbilical cord and breastmilk to newborns. In addition, developing children will naturally copy their mothers, including daily habits around consumption and self-care, so *before* conception is the opportune time to release attachments to unhealthy food and drink and to exercise regularly to develop a strong pelvic floor. Drink the best water you can source.

Consult with your physician if you are under medical treatment for a diagnosed condition

Consult with your physician before doing this fast if you are under medical treatment, especially if you have kidney disease or congestive heart issues or are taking prescription medications for high blood pressure that change how your body metabolizes potassium. Talk to your physician about your desire to fast and be prepared to get a set of directives from your physician about changing your diet, drink habits and exercise. If your physician doesn't know about these self-care practices, seek a holistic and naturopathic physician who practices detoxification to help you. Many prescribe 30-day restricted diets with a supplement regimen that supports better detoxification metabolism. If you have been diagnosed with cancer and are interested in detoxification, you will want to learn about the more rigorous Gerson Therapy or explore Chris Wark's Square One Healing Cancer Coaching Program to get your special needs met safely.

Prepare to fast by eating raw vegan organic whole foods for 2 days

To prepare to go into a fast properly, give your digestive tract two days eating raw organic vegan whole foods. Help yourself have an easy transition. Raw foods have enzymes that help us digest the food, and by eating raw you eliminate the most inflammatory and nutrient-depleted processed foods that take a lot of water to digest and eliminate, and are constipating and acidifying. If you are constipated, continue eating raw organic vegan whole foods for as many days as you need until you have a healthy bowel movement. Then start your fast. Drink plenty of the best quality water you can source—spring water or filtered alkaline water. Avoid salting your food. Too much sodium and not enough potassium will cause you to hold onto water and waste.

The daily routine: drink, move and release

You are doing four things every day while fasting. Only four. Be rigorous about them.

1. **Drink.** Hydrate and nutrient-saturate yourself by drinking nutrient-dense drinks throughout the day (recipes below).

2. **Move.** Walk vigorously 20-45 minutes outdoors every day to fire up oxygen metabolism; if the weather doesn't cooperate, exercise indoors to break a light sweat, stimulate deeper breathing, and move blood and lymph.

3. **Release.** Do a 12-minute coffee enema.

4. **Supplement.** Take Vitamin D3 with K2 in the morning and magnesium and herbal intestinal movement formula before bed. Between drinks take activated charcoal to bind waste and toxic substances and help yourself eliminate them faster. Avoid taking charcoal with your supplements, it will bind them and you'll poop them out without absorbing them.

That's it; it's the same routine for 10 days, simple, with profound effects.

The 7 daily drinks

You will drink around 4 quarts of fluids a day, depending on your body size and how dehydrated and nutrient-depleted you are. Consume all 7 nutrient-dense drinks daily to hydrate and nutrient-saturate your cells, tissues, organs and glands, and to flush toxic waste and excrement out of your body.

1 serving = 8 ounces.

1. Cold-pressed raw vegetable juices. (3 servings)
2. Superfood shakes with ground chia seeds and organic raw apple juice. (2-3 servings)
3. Potassium-rich vegetable broth served with a spoonful each of olive oil and coconut oil, and fresh ground black pepper. (2-3 servings)
4. Spicy lemonade with maple syrup or honey and cayenne pepper. (4 servings)
5. Detox tea. (2-3 servings)
6. Raw coconut water. (2 servings)
7. Kombucha. (1 serving)

Why these drinks matter

1. **Raw vegetable juices provide structured alkaline water loaded with vitamins and electrolyte minerals to hungry, thirsty cells, and provide enzymes to aid digestion, detoxification and elimination of food waste and feces.**

Juices need to be cold-pressed raw to be nutrient-dense and bioavailable. Once heated (pasteurized) the natural enzymes in them are denatured and no longer bioavailable. Those enzymes make all the difference in the world to our digestion and to elimination of waste. Stick with organic vegetables, fruits are too sugary.

2. Superfood shakes are so packed with nutrients, they act as a meal replacement.

Superfood mixes on the market today are a feat of postmodern culture. If we individually tried to source all the ingredients in them, it would cost a small fortune. Look for a superfood brand that combines plants sourced from both land and sea, as well as freshwater algae like chlorella and spirulina that pack a bioavailable dose of protein—more than a steak without all the digesting and eliminating of waste that comes with eating animal flesh. These plants are ground up, rendering the nutrients predigested and easier to absorb. When multiple nutrient-dense plant foods are combined, they become a nutrient-dense superfood mix that functions as an essential-nutrient meal replacement. When mixed with ground chia seeds loaded with omegas 3, 6, 9, they also provide essential fats. They also contain beneficial phytonutrients and often include adaptogens like aswhagandha and reishi mushroom.

There are many excellent superfood brands to choose from on the market. My personal favorite is Dr. Schulze's Superfood Plus. I like this brand because of its quality, it sells wholesale to practitioners, and because Dr. Schulze's main store is a short drive from my home in West Los Angeles. I can also buy it down the street at the local health food store. Find what is available to you locally or order online.

3. Potassium-rich vegetable broth helps us correct a common electrolyte mineral imbalance that makes it hard to hydrate and eliminate waste across cell walls.

The optimal ratio of potassium to sodium for our internal bioterrain is roughly twice as much potassium as sodium. Americans tend to have the reverse—too much sodium and not enough potassium — because we over-salt our food and use refined salt that is 100% sodium. Eating this way creates a chronic electrolyte imbalance that drinking potassium-rich vegetable broth everyday helps to remedy.

4. Spicy lemonade hydrates, alkalinizes and lowers blood pressure.

Freshly made lemonade with a spoonful of maple syrup or honey and a kick of cayenne pepper provides B vitamins, Vitamin C and capsaicin—a plant compound in cayenne that lowers blood pressure and triggers digestive enzyme production. Though acidic, lemons once digested and metabolized create alkaline byproducts that make us more alkaline.

5. Herbal detox teas contain liver-detoxifying herbs that help your liver flush waste.

Burdock root is a classic liver detoxifier, but there are many such herbs depending on geography. Chinese liver herbs are different in this respect from North American ones, but these plants are all bitter and have a similar effect on the liver, stimulating it to purge its bile and toxin-laden waste through the gallbladder and into the colon for fast elimination. The herbs also soothe the liver ducts and calm the nerves. There are many detox teas on the market. You're going to get a richer tea if you buy loose leaf brands instead of teabags. There are a multitude of good detox teas on the market, but my favorite is Dr. Schulze's Detox Tea because some of his North American herbs are wild harvested. If you suffer bladder irritation, try his Kidney-Bladder Tea.

6. Raw coconut water hydrates faster than water because it's loaded with electrolytes.

Coconut water is mineral rich. It contains calcium, magnesium and phosphorous, and packs a punch of potassium. These electrolyte minerals make coconut water quickly and deeply hydrating. It's an indulgent treat to serve yourself raw coconut water during a wet fast. By Day 5, one glass of it will taste divine.

7. Kombucha is loaded with probiotics and B vitamins.

Drinking kombucha provides some good gut bacteria and lots of B vitamins necessary for cellular energy production. Its natural fermented bubbliness is refreshing to the mouth and can help clear the palate.

Drink recipes

1. Cold-pressed vegetable juices

- If you have a juicer, juicing at home is more cost effective than buying pre-made juices. Use a cold-pressed juicer — you want the juice not the fiber.

- Carrot, beet and celery make a good base. Just drink all celery juice if you want to keep it simple. Carrot and beet are more starchy and sugary root vegetables, so avoid overconsuming them. Juice spinach, cabbage, cucumber and watercress to change it up.

- If you purchase your juices premade, buy organic, raw, cold-pressed vegetable juices off the shelf or at a juice bar. Prefer glass to plastic bottles if you have a choice.

2. Superfood shakes

- Mix a couple tablespoons of superfood powder with 16 oz. of organic raw apple juice. —Add ground chia seeds for omega 3, 6, 9 essential fats.

- Keep prep simple and shake it up by hand in a mason jar. Or prepare in a blender adding blueberries or cacao, and a dash of cinnamon.

- Serve for breakfast and lunch.

3. Potassium broth

- In a large soup pot, add 5 organic beets with beet greens, 5 carrots, 5 celery stalks, the skins of 5 potatoes (discard the potato flesh, it's too starchy), 2 onions, 10 garlic cloves, and herbs to taste (sage and thyme are my favorites).

- Cover in spring water or filtered alkaline water and simmer on low for 2-3 hrs.

- DO NOT SALT AND DO NOT BOIL. The broth will turn a deep bright red. If you boil it, it will oxidize and turn brown and you will have to throw it out and start over.

- Serve the broth warm, not hot, with fresh ground black pepper and add a spoonful each of olive oil and coconut oil for a dose of essential fats to feed your immune system, endocrine system, nervous system and gut mucosa—not to mention your skin, hair, eyes and joints.

- In hotter summer months, store the broth in the refrigerator, blend with a spoonful of olive and coconut oil before serving, and it turns a frothy beautiful hot pink color perfect to share with guests. Serve cold. Eat 2-3 servings (16 to 24 ounces) for dinner.

4. Spicy lemonade

- Squeeze 2-3 lemons into a quart of warm spring or filtered water. Meyer's lemons are best.

- Add a spoonful of maple syrup or honey for B vitamins and a stiff shake or two of cayenne pepper for capsaicin. Stir it up.

- Drop some rind in, as lemon peel is full of Vitamin C, fiber and small amounts of calcium, magnesium and potassium.

- Serve hot or cold. It's a good drink to start the morning with.

5. Detox tea

- Buy detox tea in bulk rather than in tea bags to get a full rich tea extract of the herbs.

- Put 2 or 3 tablespoons of herbal tea in a medium-sized pot of spring or filtered water and soak for at least 20 minutes. Overnight is better.

- Bring to a boil, reduce to simmer, and simmer for 20-30 minutes.

- A pot of hot detox tea simmering on your stove will fill your kitchen with a heart-warming smell that calms the nerves when you walk in the house.

6. Coconut water

- Buy whole coconuts and use a compostable straw to skip the plastic bottles, if you can source whole coconuts and know how to open them safely.
- Or buy raw, unpasteurized coconut water brands off the shelf. Health food stores and juice bars usually carry raw coconut water if you can't find it at your local grocer, though most supermarket chains carry it now.

7. Kombucha

- You can make your own kombucha with a starter mushroom and a glass cannister. Add green tea and sugar to feed the mushroom. Cover and set away in a dark corner to ferment.
- Bottled kombucha is easily available to purchase these days and there's plenty of brands to choose from.

4 supplements to help eliminate waste faster

Take these 4 supplements every day during your fast to optimize detoxification and elimination of waste and feces during fasting, and to bolster stronger immune function.

1. Vitamin D3 with K2 (in the morning)
2. Activated charcoal (on an empty stomach)
3. Magnesium (before bed)
4. Herbal intestinal movement formula (before bed)

Why these supplements matter

During fasting we expel acidic waste out of cells, tissues and organs, so we want to metabolize, collect and excrete our waste faster than we make it—or at least as fast as we make it—to prevent feeling congested, toxic and "shitty" as we commonly say for a reason. It's a body metaphor we all understand.

If your body does the opposite—makes waste faster than you can excrete it—you might find yourself in a foul mood pacing around in circles until you get your toxic waste out. Until you do, you may feel irritable, achy, headachy, tired and foggy. Those are signals that you need to hydrate and move more to help yourself eliminate your own waste faster. If you haven't done your coffee enema, now is the time. If you've already done a coffee enema, feel free to do another one (coffee enema instructions below.)

Here's what each supplement does for you during your fast to help you metabolize, detoxify and eliminate waste more effectively.

Vitamin D3 with K2 strengthens immunity, increases intestinal absorption and supports healthy bone density

Taking a daily supplement of 5000 IU Vitamin D3 with Vitamin K2 supports the intestinal absorption of calcium, magnesium and phosphate, regulates cell growth, increases intestinal absorption of nutrients, and supports bone growth and bone density. Choose a brand that combines Vitamin D3 with Vitamin K2 because K2 helps your body deliver calcium to your bones and teeth instead of floating around in your bloodstream clogging up your arteries.

My favorite brand is Designs for Health D-Evail highly bioavailable vitamin D with K1, K2 and GG. These are gel caps and I feel I absorb them better than a powdered supplement. Based on my annual hormone blood analysis, I need 5,000 to 10,000 IU of Vitamin D daily, and I live in the Southern California sunshine with a beach to walk on and a roof deck for sunning even in winter. Why do I still need to supplement with Vitamin D? Because my mother is Filipino and she and her ancestors lived in the tropics. Many of them were fishermen out in the sun every day. Those are my genes.

Vitamin D also plays a critical role in immunity by providing a metabolite that our liver uses to metabolize markers for our immune system, known as glycoprotein Macrophage Activating Factor (gMAF). Without gMAF, white blood cell macrophages will float by not knowing to respond to a pathogen like a bacterium or virus, or to a damaged or cancerous cell. Our body needs an abundant supply of Vitamin D, oleic acid (olive oil is full of oleic acid) and testosterone to make these immune markers.

Even if you supplement with an oral Vitamin D supplement, it's a good practice to get sun directly on your skin every day that you can while fasting so you can make your own Vitamin D—the best kind. Your skin will love you for sunbathing, even if it's just 20 minutes sipping a cup of hot tea or spicy lemonade in a chair set by a sunny window. Full body sunbathing on a warm sunny day is even better. Sunshine on your skin also triggers melanin production in your pineal gland—a precursor to melatonin that regulates our circadian rhythm and sleep cycle. If you suffer from insomnia, get more sunshine for more Vitamin D and melanin. It will help you reset your internal clock to sleep at night and wake up in the morning, rather than stay up at night and sleep in.

Activated charcoal binds to toxic waste so you can eliminate it faster

Many supplement brands offer an activated charcoal. You can find it at health food stores and whole foods markets, and even at chain drugstores. My favorite is Bulletproof Activated Charcoal. I always have it on my shelf. And always travel with some.

Activated charcoal helps remove heavy metals like mercury, aluminum and lead, and binds with toxins derived from urea, the by-product of protein digestion. Take 1 or 2 capsules—always on an empty stomach. Avoid taking charcoal with anything else, such as supplements or superfood, because charcoal will bind minerals and other nutrients and you'll end up pooping them out with your charcoal and wasting your money.

If you're worried about mercury amalgam dental fillings in your teeth (the silver ones, though they often turn blackish gray over time), you can open a capsule of charcoal into your mouth. Chew it a bit to get it moist, but don't swallow. Hold it in your mouth for several minutes to give it time to bind with mercury, and then spit it out. *(Tip: don't spit it out in your sink, it can stop it up.)*

Magnesium hydrates, calms and opens the colon

Magnesium is an electrolyte mineral essential for proper cell hydration that most Americans lack in sufficient amounts to sustain their health. It's one of the most common nutrient deficiencies among modern humans that rely on industrial agriculture, which strips minerals from the soil over time. Magnesium is essential for over 600 metabolic chemical reactions in our body, including over 300 enzyme reactions, many of them taking place in our gut and liver.

There are many good brands of magnesium supplements to choose from. One of my tried-and-true cost-effective favorites is Magnesium Calm, a magnesium powder you mix with warm water that tastes like raspberry or citrus. If you're willing to spend a little more, check out Eidon Ionic Minerals Magnesium to enjoy highly bioavailable magnesium in de-ionized water for better absorption. You can also put magnesium salts in a hot bath to soak magnesium in through your skin. It's a lovely way to get your magnesium and prepare for a good night's sleep if you struggle with insomnia. If you don't have time for a bath, rub a handful of magnesium salts on your skin around your kidneys, liver and belly in a hot shower. *(Tip: install a shower filter or bath ball filter to clean your bathing water of chlorine, chloramine, fluoride and other toxic substances in tap water in many cities.)*

Getting enough magnesium daily can trigger dramatic changes in your health and moods, because magnesium is essential for healthy nerve transmission and neuromuscular coordination, and it protects nerve cells from excitotoxicity (stress). Magnesium is also essential for making happy, balanced feel-good hormones. It affects concentrations of parathyroid hormone and the active form of Vitamin D (hormone D) that regulate bone homeostasis. Magnesium calms the nervous system by regulating the HPA-axis hormones in response to stress (hypothalamus, pituitary, adrenal). It also normalizes insulin, reduces blood sugar and has a laxative effect on the colon.

Intestinal movement formulas help excrete stool and soothe the gut mucosa

Taking a capsule or two of herbal intestinal movement formula with a cup of detox tea every evening before bed primes some good bowel movements in the morning. There are many good brands to choose from. My favorite is Health Force Intestinal Movement Formula because of its gentle effectiveness.

If you've been over-consuming, eating too much cooked and processed foods that have created a lot of waste over time, you can accumulate a layer of fecal plaque lining your intestines and colon. An intestinal movement formula of detoxifying and soothing herbs helps break that plaque up, move it out and soothe the mucosal lining of the intestines, colon and rectum. Unlike synthetic laxatives sold by the pharmaceutical industry such as MiraLax that comes with a FDA warning label for propylene glycol, herbal intestinal movement formulas are natural, gentle and safe.

Coffee enemas—getting down and dirty on waste elimination

We need to talk shit about the waste management problem Americans have created because of our economy of mass consumerism that has driven generations of overconsumption and created the inevitable toxic waste that comes of it. For people who have done enemas before and use them as a staple of their self-care practices, talking about coffee enemas is like talking about drinking enough water. Of course we need to drink water and of course we need to eliminate our own waste efficiently. However, for those who haven't done enemas before, there are generally two psychological responses: one is curiosity and the other is resistance. Resistance feels like closed doors, window blinds drawn, end of conversation. Suddenly there's a blockage, resistance and even repugnance, as if our colon, rectum and anus are parts of us we don't want to talk about, much less touch and care for. Let's not think about our waste, much less talk about how to manage it! is the vibration.

Coffee enemas provide a critical somatic feedback loop to help you self-regulate your own attachments to overconsumption and too much waste—about what you're putting in your mouth, how much and how often, and what is coming out the other end—or not coming out the other end—because of it. In a culture of overconsumption where people are accustomed to flushing their toxic waste down the toilet for someone else to deal with, doing a coffee enema can be psychologically liberating. It's a sobering reality check that we all need from time to time. And it's also, divinely, a fast remedy when combined with a few days of fasting from eating food. Our body delights in feeling clean and empty, yet hydrated and nutrient saturated with plenty of fresh air and sunshine on our skin and in our eyes when we take a walk in nature. It feels so good to be alive.

It doesn't feel good to sit in a chair constipated and dehydrated day after day while eating and eating. As animals we are tuned in our DNA to be either moving, eating, sleeping or connecting. Which means if we're not moving enough, sleeping enough and connecting enough, we're eating more. You're not running if you're chewing, and you're not chewing if you're running. And you're not eating if you're talking, and if you are you want to change that habit right now to improve your digestive health and clear your mind.

There's a gravity to ignoring the impulse to stand up to breathe and take a walk in the sun to activate some feel-good messenger hormones, stimulate faster metabolism by sucking in more oxygen and exhaling more CO_2 for optimal gas exchange with your blood, help your pumping heart ease its load, and trigger peristalsis to move food and food waste out of the intestines and feces out of the colon. Taking a walk clears your head. Constipation makes you foggy because it fills your blood with your own toxic acidic waste and stresses out your heart. It feels depressing.

Coffee enemas during 10 days of fasting changes all that fast.

I've seen everything from dark brown slimy fecal plaque to greenish gallstones to yellowish candida fungus in the toilet after coffee enemas. And more waste than I thought possible. What I can say to those of you who are curious about coffee enemas is that those direct experiences I've had with my body's waste impacted my sense of my embodied self and my self-care, and forever changed my attachments to the foods and drinks that I, and I alone, put in my mouth.

Let's be frank. Around their anus and rectum is where a lot of people experience emotional blockages. Feelings of repugnance, nervous laughter, silly jokes, not to mention fear and disgust, constipated inertia or explosive anger. It could sound like *"What? Not me! That's disgusting! I'm not doing that!"*

Do your daily coffee enema while you're fasting! It is a core component of Fast Therapy because it takes you faster than anything else to the core of your attachments to consumption and waste. And that will set you up for some fast therapy for the 10 days of your fast.

By the way, if you're a coffee lover and you've never done a coffee enema before, you have a real treat in store for you. IT'S A REAL WAKE UP CALL! Just be aware if you do one at night, you'll be awake and energized afterward.

How coffee enemas work

Your colon and rectum absorb water from feces before excretion to regulate water loss. The exception is diarrhea when you urgently need to purge poisons, toxic substances and/or bad bacteria from rotten food as fast as possible, and that's why diarrhea comes with a risk of dehydration if it goes on too long.

When you put coffee into your rectum, the coffee gets absorbed into your descending colon and then into your liver through a system of drainage ducts through which your liver dumps the waste it has collected from filtering digested food particles through your gut mucosa and also filtering your blood. If you're eating a lot and the food you're eating is full of acidic sugars and toxic substances, it can be a lot of very acidic and toxic waste. Coffee enemas are basically a way to backflush this drainage and reabsorption system. It's a way to address the problem at its root and help you feel better fast.

The effect of coffee on your liver is immediate. By a divine act of nature, palmitate enzymes in coffee trigger the liver to secrete glutathione—three to four times the amount of glutathione it usually secretes. Glutathione is an enzyme known as the mother of all antioxidants that we metabolize ourselves in our liver. It is the key enzyme for detoxification because of the role it plays in cleaning dirty genes and breaking down waste so it can be eliminated from the body faster and more effectively. And, icing on the cake, acids in coffee help break down fecal plaque along the mucosal lining of the descending colon and rectum so it can be flushed out of the body.

Because of the detoxifying effects on the liver and colon, a coffee enema is a self-care tool that can stop a toxic headache in its tracks.

It can help you relieve constipation, and it can clear your head and get you back in the groove with energy for life. If you feel icky or achy during a fast because toxic waste is being released faster than you can eliminate it, do your coffee enema and feel better 12 minutes later. It's that simple and that fast.

Coffee enema instructions

1. Organic coffee (mold and fungicide free).

2. Disposable Fleet enema bottle (large size) or reusable latex enema bag available online or at any drugstore. If you're using a disposable Fleet enema bottle, discard the saline solution and rinse before adding warm coffee.

After a morning bowel movement is a good time to do a coffee enema. But any time you feel foggy and sluggish and need relief is a good time.

Boil 2 to 4 tablespoons of organic ground coffee on the stove with 16-20 ounces of clean distilled, spring or filtered water. Or make a very strong pot of coffee in a French press.

Let the coffee cool down to your body temperature. Avoid too hot or too cold. If you only have so much time and can't wait for the coffee to cool naturally, you can make your coffee solution extra strong and then add cool water to it.

Pour 1-4 cups of warm coffee into your enema bottles or bag, depending on your body size and size of your descending colon. Colons under chronic stress can become enlarged and distended in an attempt to hold more waste. You'll have a sense of how much you can hold.

Lubricate the nozzle with a little coconut oil, lie down comfortably on your left side if you're right-handed, relax, and gently insert the nozzle into your rectum. Squeeze your fleet enema bottle or release the clasp on an enema bag suspended above you to put the coffee into your rectum. Roll onto your left side (descending colon is on the left) for a couple minutes to help the coffee get absorbed from your rectum into your colon, then roll onto your right side to help the coffee get absorbed from your colon into your liver which is on the right. You might hear and feel some gurgling in your liver.

Hold the coffee in for 12 minutes (or as long as you can). After 12 minutes, get up and let everything go in the toilet. And flush away.

Alternatives to coffee enemas

Okay, that's my coffee enema spiel. Thanks for listening. If you're still not convinced, I give you two alternative options below that provide similar effects.

But honestly, neither of these options are as good psychologically or physically as doing a daily coffee enema yourself, or as healing for someone who is carrying a lot of waste from chronic overconsumption and chronic constipation. Dealing with your own waste is eye-opening to say the least. However, you can do Fast Therapy and get good results with these alternatives.

Alternative 1: Schedule a session or two with a colon hydrotherapist during your 10-day fast to let a professional help you flush toxic waste and fecal plaque from your liver, colon and rectum. Day 3 and Day 8 are ideal. Ask your colon hydrotherapist to add coffee to your colonic. You can also ask for chlorophyll or ozonated water to bring oxygen therapy into your colonic as well. Colon hydrotherapists tend to be practical people who are down to earth about waste management and nutrition. They naturally want to talk to you during your colonic about healthy lifestyle changes you could make to help yourself be more well. What they say to you may catch your attention and have more impact than usual because you'll be watching your own feces and waste coming out of a clear drainage tube while they're talking to you about what you've been eating!

Alternate 2: Buy a liposomal glutathione supplement and pump 2 or 3 squirts in your mouth daily during your fast, holding it on your tongue for 30 seconds before swallowing to get a dose of this powerful antioxidant enzyme to support faster methylation, detoxification and elimination of waste. Liposomal delivery makes the glutathione more bioavailable. I use Quicksilver Scientific's liposomal glutathione for its quality and glass bottle, designed by detox chemist Dr. Christopher Shade to be used as part of his heavy metal detox kit. By the way, if you really want to get your waste out fast because you are concerned about a high toxic bioburden, squirt some glutathione in your mouth AND do a coffee enema.

What if you don't do any of these options?

Can you do the 10-day nutritional wet fast without doing coffee enemas or taking liposomal glutathione orally or getting a colonic? I don't recommend this, but I know it happens. The father struggling with high blood pressure whose testimony I shared didn't do a coffee enema, colonic or glutathione supplementation, and he *still* had an optimal blood pressure reading on Day 10, lost 7 lbs. in fat burn and waste elimination, and felt transformed physically, emotionally and spiritually. However, he also reported that he struggled through the experience. Had he done his coffee enemas, he would have liberated himself from a lot of the struggle. Skipping the coffee enemas is the hard way to do this fast. The faster you eliminate your waste from your body, the better you feel.

Fasting mantras

Whenever you feel challenged during your fast, repeat these three mantras to help yourself stay focused.

1. My discipline is my freedom.
2. My journey is my destination.
3. My body knows the truth.

Planning tools

Use the visual guides on the following pages to get organized to fast: two-week overview, daily schedule, shopping list, recipes, dailytracker.

Once you dive into your fast, start the daily embodied therapy sessions in Part Three for some Fast Therapy.

FAST THERAPY
2-Week Overview

RAW VEGAN	**RAW VEGAN**	**01** FAST	**02** FAST
03 FAST	**04** FAST	**05** FAST	**06** FAST
07 FAST	**08** FAST	**09** FAST	**10** FAST
RAW VEGAN	**RAW VEGAN**		

FAST THERAPY
Daily Fasting Schedule

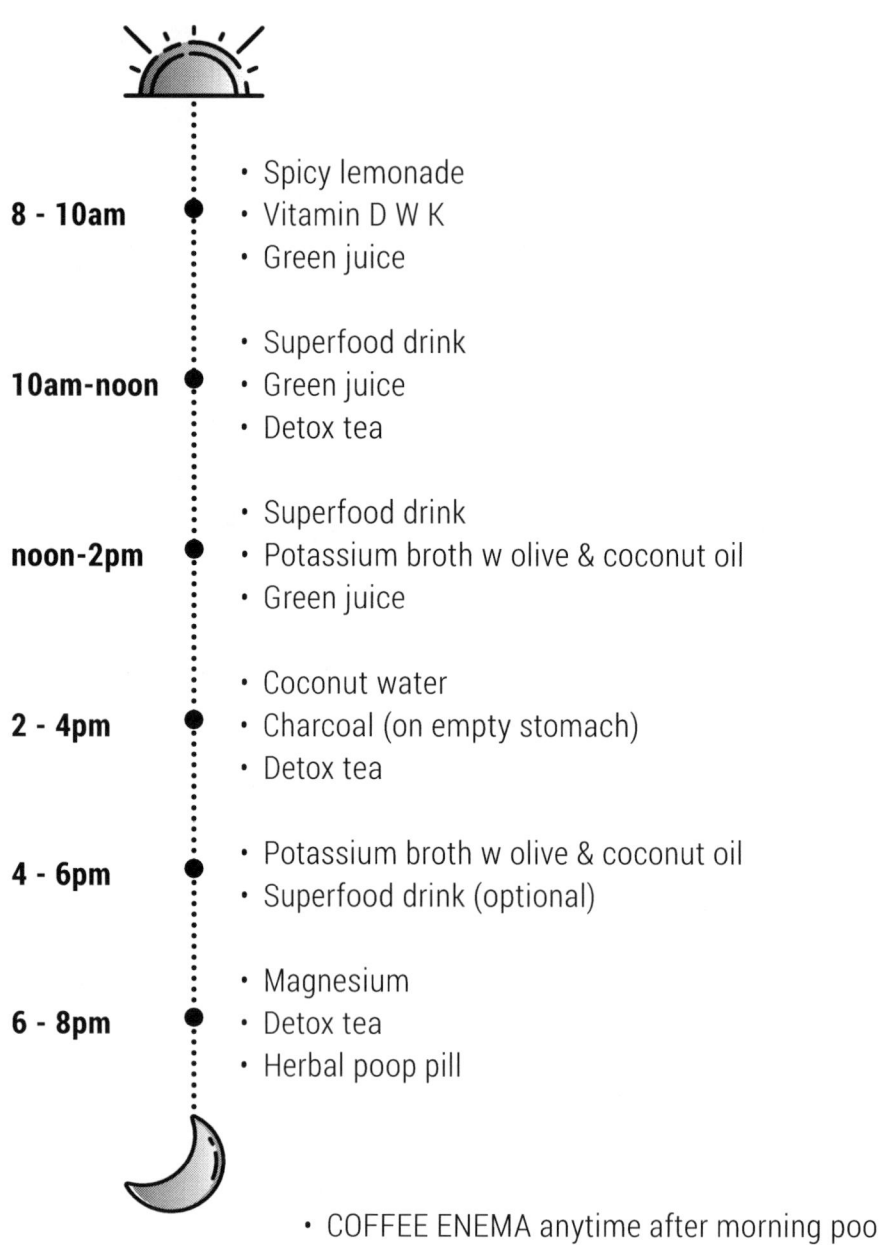

8 - 10am
- Spicy lemonade
- Vitamin D W K
- Green juice

10am-noon
- Superfood drink
- Green juice
- Detox tea

noon-2pm
- Superfood drink
- Potassium broth w olive & coconut oil
- Green juice

2 - 4pm
- Coconut water
- Charcoal (on empty stomach)
- Detox tea

4 - 6pm
- Potassium broth w olive & coconut oil
- Superfood drink (optional)

6 - 8pm
- Magnesium
- Detox tea
- Herbal poop pill

- COFFEE ENEMA anytime after morning poo
- WALK IN NATURE 20-45 min daily

FAST THERAPY
Shopping List

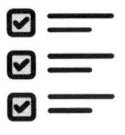

Everything you need for 10 days:

DRINKS

- **For superfood shakes:**
  1 container superfood powder (14oz)
  1.5 - 2 gallons of raw apple juice
  1 package ground chia seeds
  Blueberries or cacao optional

- **For 3 batches of potassium broth:**
  6 onions, 15 potatoes, 15 carrots, 15 beets w/ greens, 15 celery stalks, 30 garlic cloves, fresh black pepper, virgin coconut oil & olive oil

- **For raw juices:**
  2-3 bunches celery, 2-3 bunches carrots, 2-3 bunches spinach or chard, 30 apples, 10 cucumbers, 1 large ginger root.

- **For spicy lemonade:**
  20-30 lemons, maple syrup or honey, cayenne pepper.

- **Detox tea:**
  1 bag loose leaf herbal tea (16oz) or 2 boxes of tea bags for 30 servings.

- **Raw coconut water:**
  10 coconuts, or five 32oz bottles for ten 16 oz servings.

SUPPLEMENTS

- Herbal Intestinal Movement Formula
- Activated Charcoal
- Magnesium supplement
- Vitamin D w K (5000 IU)

COFFEE ENEMAS

- Fleet enema bottle or reusabe enema bag
- Organic ground coffee (preferably dark roast)

FAST THERAPY
Recipes

Everything you need for 10 days:

2 servings daily | **For your superfood shake:**
Mix 2 tbsp of raw green superfood mix with some organic, unfiltered apple juice and water in a jar, add 1-2 tbsp of chia seeds, shake and drink up for a potent dose of vitamins, minerals, phytonutrients, enzymes and antioxidants. Remember those chia seeds for good omegas 3-6-9 because they will help you feel full and suppress your appetite.

3 servings daily | **For your raw veggie juice:**
Raw means unpasteurized. Other than apple juice which makes veggies more digestible, stay away from sugary fruit juices and stick with vegetables like carrots, beets, celery, cabbage, broccoli and cucumber, and dark leafy greens like spinach and chard. Add ginger or garlic to spice it up.

2-3 servings daily | **For your potassium broth:**
Skin of 5 potatoes (discard the potato flesh, it's too starchy), 5 beets, 5 carrots, 5 celery stalks, 2 onions, 10 garlic cloves. Cover in a gallon of filtered water in a big soup pot and simmer for 1-3 hours (it should be a bright red). DO NOT BOIL. DO NOT SALT. Sodium causes cell and organ membranes to close, and we're trying to open them. Serve the broth with a spoonful of coconut oil, a spoonful of olive oil, and fresh ground black pepper.

FAST THERAPY
Daily Tracker: Days 1-5

Check off each item for each day to track your progress:

DAILY NUTRIENTS & SUPPLEMENTS		1	2	3	4	5
Spicy Lemonade	1 qt /32 oz.					
Detox Tea	3 servings /24 oz.					
Potassium Broth	2-3 servings /16-24 oz.					
Raw Green Juice	3 servings /24 oz.					
Coconut Water	2 servings /16 oz.					
Superfood Drink	2-3 servings /16-24 oz.					
Coffee Enema						
Vitamin D w K						
Charcoal Binder						
Magnesium						
Herbal Poop Pill						

FAST THERAPY
Daily Tracker: Days 6-10

Check off each item for each day to track your progress:

DAILY NUTRIENTS & SUPPLEMENTS		6	7	8	9	10
Spicy Lemonade	1 qt /32 oz.					
Detox Tea	3 servings /24 oz.					
Potassium Broth	2-3 servings /16-24 oz.					
Raw Green Juice	3 servings /24 oz.					
Coconut Water	2 servings /16 oz.					
Superfood Drink	2 servings /16 oz.					
Coffee Enema						
Vitamin D w K						
Charcoal Binder						
Magnesium						
Herbal Poop Pill						

FASTING Q & A

Fasting for women—carb cravings

Nutritional wet fasting helps women fast long enough to see and feel the difference by providing optimal nutritional support. Women often have trouble fasting because hormonal fluctuations can drive food cravings—translated by the food industry into carb cravings. However, if you don't work by the sweat of your brow and you're not a long-distance biker, runner, mountain climber, swimmer, surfer or buff gym rat, it's not carbs you're really wanting. It's good fats and proteins, along with vegetable-sourced vitamins, minerals and phytonutrients we all need to live healthily and happily in our embodiment.

> **Takeaway:** *nutritional wet fasting enables women to feed their body the essential nutrients they need to stabilize hormones and balance blood sugar while fasting, starve candida fungus in the gut that lives on sugar and processed carbs, and eliminate neurotoxic waste from candida die-off.*

Can I fast if I'm on my period?

Menstruation is part of our detoxification system; it's how women detoxify their uterus. Fasting can help you cleanse, nutrient saturate and restore your reproductive organs.

> **Takeaway:** *you can fast on your period if you need too; though many women prefer to avoid mixing apples and oranges, since there's already a lot of action going on in the detoxification and elimination department during fasting days.*

Do I have to fast for all 10 days?

You will feel and see positive cleansing benefits in as little as 3 days of fasting. You'll get better results if you fast for 5-7 days in terms of metabolism, detoxification, elimination of waste and fat burn. However, 10 days is optimal, because the biggest changes occur between Days 8-10. If you have a difficult start, please remember that every day that goes by it gets easier. If you make it to Day 3 it's easier to make it to Day 5, if you can make it to Day 5 it's even easier to make it to Day 7, and if you make it to Day 7, from there it's even easier to make it to Day 10. Do your best to stay in the flow and reap the full benefits.

Takeaway: *you will miss the best part of this fast if you get through the first 3 days and then give up. The longer you stay in, the better results you'll get.*

Will I starve?

If you've been eating poorly and having trouble digesting and absorbing your food and eliminating the waste, you may get more bioavailable essential nutrients on this nutritional wet fast than you get eating three meals a day of nutrient-depleted cooked and processed foods and snacking in between. Still, I understand that fears can surface around the thought of not eating food. If you tend to fret over your next meal or snack when you are actually habitually overconsuming food, take some good advice from wilderness survival coach Jessie Krebs. Krebs reminds her trainees that humans in a survival situation can go about 30 days without food—at least 3 weeks even if injured—as long as water is available. She also cautions that eating and digesting food requires a lot of water, and for this reason, if you're dehydrated, eating food will only make you more dehydrated. *"Water is more important than food,"* she says, *"you're not as hungry as you think you are. It really is a mental game. Our physiology is built for fasting."*

Takeaway: *if you want to fret and worry over something while fasting, worry about drinking your daily drinks rather than eating.*

How is this fast different from intermittent fasting?

Intermittent fasting which is trending these days is also known as time-restricted eating because you restrict your consumption of food to an 8-hour window every day—typically from 10am to 6pm, or 9am to 5pm. It's like daily micro-fasting. When you restrict eating to an 8-hour window, you leave yourself 16 hours to channel water, energy and resources into detoxification, waste elimination, hormone regulation, and immunity. Less digestion of food leaves more time for everything else. For this reason, intermittent fasting can be transformative for people who habitually overconsume food and drink from the crack of dawn until they collapse into bed at night.

The primary difference between intermittent fasting and a nutritional wet fast is that the time you abstain from consuming, eating and digesting food is measured in hours vs. days. Nutritional wet fasting is a bigger slice of time, and so it produces bigger results faster. There is another payoff for giving up eating solid food for 10 days rather than for 16 hours a day (8 of which you are asleep): when it's over you feel far more detached from habitual patterns of consumption.

Takeaway: *nutritional fasting produces bigger results faster in terms of weight loss, fat burn and waste elimination. Intermittent fasting is a great way to transition back to eating cooked food after a 10-day nutritional wet fast. It keeps the ball rolling toward better gut health and keeps a lid on overconsumption.*

When to start the 10 daily embodied therapy sessions

When you start Day 1 of your fast, start the therapy sessions in Part Three to turn your fast into Fast Therapy. If you are a habitual speed reader addicted to fast consumption and scanning the surface for insights that jump out at you without necessarily ingesting all the details, you might be tempted to speed read ahead even though you haven't even started fasting.

You can do that. The words will be the same. However, **you** will be different. If you haven't started to fast yet, stand up on your own two feet, gather your parts and go shopping for what you need, dive into the fast, and come back here later. If you're with me and you're in your fast, start with Session 1.

Complete one session a day

The sessions start in your mouth and end at your feet and cover everything else in between. Complete one session a day for each day of your 10-day fast. If you let yourself be satisfied with one session a day, you will give yourself time to digest and absorb each lesson and set of exercises before you move forward. I encourage you to give your embodied consciousness time to shift to get the most impact with longer lasting effects. If you break the sequence because you fall behind or because one of the later sessions has your name written all over it and you skip forward because you just can't help yourself, or you need fast support and guidance for that part of you that is hurting or struggling, that's okay. But finish all 10 sessions before the end of your 10-day fast.

PART 3
THERAPY

DAY 1 MOUTHPEACE

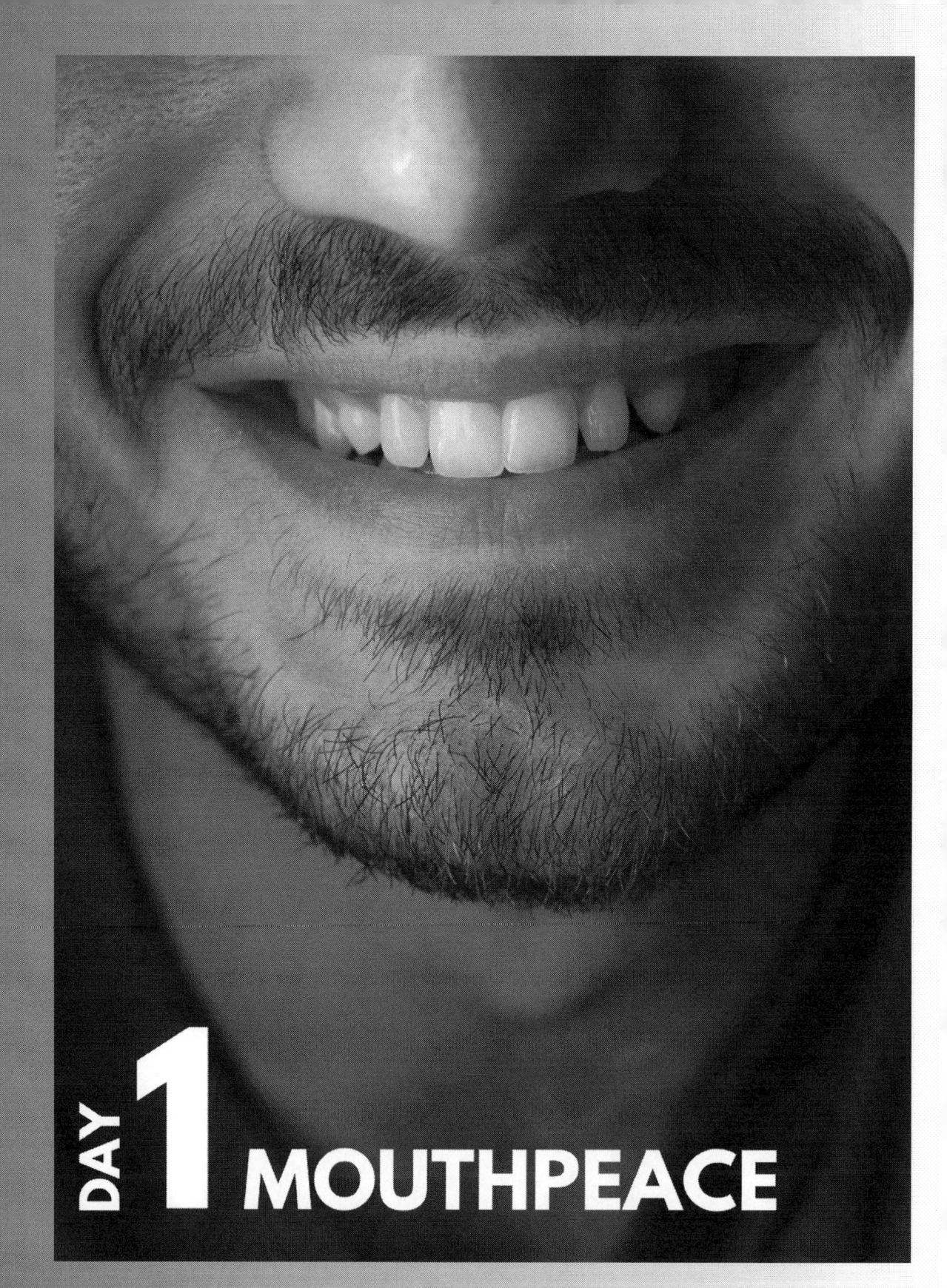

Chapter 4

MOUTHPEACE — Session One

Day 1 of the fast

Today your attention will naturally be focused on the daily routine—the 7 daily drinks, the daily coffee enema, and taking the daily supplements (Vitamin D, charcoal binder, magnesium, intestinal movement formula.) Master the routine today because it's the same simple routine for the next 9 days. The only thing that changes is you. Starting with your experience of time. When you fast, you realize how much time you spend sourcing, prepping and cooking three meals a day and snacking in between. Even eating at restaurants takes time, and money. Today you have an opportunity to use the time you save to turn your fast into Fast Therapy by doing this self-therapy session for better bodymind integration. This first session starts in your mouth, the last session ends with your feet, and in the middle we touch all your parts in between.

While your emotional and psychological attachments to food and drink will be front and center in your consciousness today in terms of what goes into your mouth as an organ of consumption, the lesson and exercises in this session nudge you to bring peace to your mouth in terms of what's coming out of it as an organ of speech. The two are connected.

Mouthbody care during fasting

Birch xylitol kills candida fungus in your gut and also kills caries bacteria in your mouth that eat away at your teeth and periodontal bacteria that feed on your gums. These microbes eat the xylitol made from the bark of birch trees but cannot digest it, causing a die-off. Every day of your fast, get up in the morning and scrape your tongue with a tongue scraper or spoon. Your tongue will detox a film of whitish mucus every night; you want to scrape that off and get it out rather than swallow it down.

After you tongue scrape, put a teaspoon of xylitol in your mouth, let it dissolve, swish for 2 minutes, then spit it out. Swishing longer isn't better; however, swishing multiple times a day does improve results. An article published in the *Journal of the American Dental Association* recommends xylitol swishing for 2 minutes 5 times a day. Or you can buy a toothpaste with xylitol. You can also buy xylitol gum. If you have concerns about your systemic mouthbody health in regard to mercury amalgam dental fillings, root canals, wisdom teeth, gum disease, etc., see my book *Mouthbody Care: Top Dental Issues that Compromise Your Health and What You Can Do about Them.*

GETTING A GRIP ON YOUR MOUTH

What you consume and what you say, what you take into your mouth and ingest and what comes out of your mouth in speech, directly affect your health and moods — including the feeling of being at peace with yourself and with others. All of us feel immediately empowered when we come to peace with the choices we make about what goes in and comes out of our mouth. Because of the mouthbody connection, without feeling peace in your mouth, it will be very difficult to create sustainable bodymind health that lasts.

Fasting brings peace to our mouth as an organ of consumption for eating and drinking. For a precious ten days, the time it takes to cleanse, restore and reset, we become more conscious about our need to consume. Learning to take a break from consumption is critical for anyone living in a consumer culture, because to a great extent our big mouths got us into our postmodern condition of chronic bodymind illnesses in the first place. With industrial technologies of mass production, we modern humans opened our mouths to constant consumption and became gaping black holes of insatiable desire. We voraciously consume and overconsume everything, and as a result we have laid waste to precious resources and created mountains and rivers and oceans of toxic waste and garbage that poison us and every other creature on the planet.

Now armed with digital communication technologies, our big mouths have become cosmic loudspeakers for all kinds of negativity and projections blocking change and stoking fires between stakeholders who, despite their differences, share a stake in a sustainable future that liberates everyone from chronic mental and physical ill health and emotional distress. What better time than fasting, when we come to peace with our mouth as an organ of consumption, to also find peace with our mouth as an organ of speech.

Habitual negativity

Habitual negative language — the kind that is unconscious and pervasive — makes it almost impossible for people around you to hear you say 'NO' when it really matters, because they hear you saying 'NO' all the time to everything. For this reason, it feels somatically, emotionally, mentally and spiritually liberating to clear unconscious negative language from your mouth during a fast. Letting go of negativity in your mouth uplifts you and everyone around you, because it makes for far more effective communication about people's actual needs.

If *'NO'* is the first thing out of your mouth as a habit, you might be challenged by the exercises in this session. You may find yourself speechless at first. But as you practice positive language, you'll find better words to express what you are observing, feeling, sensing, thinking, wanting and needing. These are positive words that feel more authentic and attractive because they are free of the constraints that negativity puts on you and the people around you.

Removing negative language from your mouth changes the vibration and tone in a room fast. It can bring peace into a house or an office in days. It can renew intimacy between lovers in trouble because positive language has a palpable somatic-emotional effect on you and the people you relate to and connect with. The benefits of purging negative language from your mouth are so profound because positivity is more than the opposite of negativity. Positivity is everything that negativity tries to negate. Positivity is pure potentiality.

Body metaphors

The body metaphors we use to describe the connections among our mouth, speech, moods and behaviors notably refer to what's coming out the other end of our gastrointestinal tract, because the two orifices are connected. *"Don't mind him, he's full of shit!"* we hear about someone running around in circles causing a ruckus seemingly looking for a place to dump his crap. Or we hear *"what an asshole!"* about a person who is agitated and acting out, again, and this time at a birthday party. Or we say that person is a *"party pooper."* When someone expresses a mountain of negative thoughts and words, we say *"what a load of crap!"* and walk away. And when someone's language is nonsensically negative and resistant to change, we say *"cut the bullshit."* That last phrase is usually stated with the person's name.

"Cut the bullshit, Camilla."

Let's face it, habitual negativity coming out of anyone's mouth is depressing. It feels like being trapped and finding yourself at a dead end. *"NOTHING WILL CHANGE!"* negativity says. And there's a suffering that comes with saying NO to everything in life. No matter how much the glass is more than half full, you and everyone around you will feel a lack of abundance when NO, NOT and NEVER are the first words out of your mouth.

Granted, there may be times in our lives when we need to say 'NO' and mean it with all our heart. Saying 'NO' to injustice for example. However, when you have that need, putting forth a solution or a remedy quickly to accentuate what you DO want will have immediate pragmatic effects on what happens next. With practice, you eventually realize you can skip the 'NO' entirely and go straight to stating the positive outcome you really want to get better results and feel better while getting them.

Benefits of positive language

The reason positive language is liberating has to do with the grammar of negativity in English and other romance languages. It's worth noting that some languages do not have a negative grammar, such as the Hopi language. Can you imagine a language in which the word 'NOT' doesn't even exist? Probably not! Because if you try to negate a negative with another negation word, the NOTs quickly proliferate. Negative grammar traps us all in a world of NOs that get attached to all the things we want and turns them into things we don't want.

Positive language, in contrast, has a liberating effect on your thoughts, moods and actions. You'll quickly notice that positive words without all the negation tend to attract positive responses. They activate feel-good hormones that have a holistic impact on you and the people in your life. Positive words are easier for people around you to understand, connect with, empathize with and talk to, because they feel like walking through doorways of possibility rather than walking down one long corridor of closed doors leading nowhere.

Somatic and psychological effects of negativity

Let's look at some examples of the way negative statements affect our emotional bodymind.

"You can't eat any food during a wet fast" is a negation of eating food. It states exactly what you don't want during a fast (eat food) and then negates that (eat food /not). Linguistically, it evokes an image of what you don't want and puts a red circle with a crossbar on top of it.

Compare the mood and vibration of the negating statement *"you can't eat any food during your fast"* to the positive statement *"drink before you're hungry."* The positive statement is a liberation from hunger rather than a negation of eating. Which feels better?

My favorite example that demonstrates the way negative statements affect us somatically and psychologically happened in a crowded power yoga class many years ago with some 80 plus people down on our mats with sweat dripping off our faces. On this Sunday morning, our guru Bryan Kest was teaching abroad, and we had a new substitute teacher we had never seen before, and honestly, never saw again. Fifteen minutes into the class, he said, *"Do this asana next, and when you do it don't look at the person's butt in front of you."*

Guess what happened? Yup. That's right. Nearly everyone, including myself. We all looked at the butt of the person in front of us. To help us maintain our concentration during what can best be described as intensely challenging sweaty yoga classes in a jam-packed dancehall, we had been trained by Bryan Kest to keep our eyes focused on the floor, the wall, or even better, outer space. One negative statement completely changed our behavior.

And then a second thing happened.

As if an ocean wave had passed through the room, everyone became self-conscious about what their butt might look like, sprawled as we were on all fours with one leg stretched out behind and one arm stretched out in front as far as we could reach. Some people responded by stretching even further into the pose, like peacocks spreading their feathers, as if a camera or spotlight had been turned on them. It was West LA. The class was full of actors. But many others visibly shrank into themselves with self-consciousness. Some just lost their concentration and began to fall out of the pose.

The flow of our flow yoga was breached. The trance broken. Soon enough thoughts like *"How much longer is this class going to last?"* and *"Who is this guy?"* began to emerge in people's minds. It was all visible in body language, as 80 pairs of eyes popped up like satellite dishes, as Bryan Kest used to describe it, to look around the room. A lot of people started giggling.

It was exactly what the new teacher *didn't* want!

Here's another example of negative language that's pertinent right now. If you think and say you can't go 10 days without eating food, you won't be able to do the 10-day nutritional wet fast or do Fast Therapy. However, if you think and say *"Yes, I can do a nutritional wet fast for 10 days and complete 10 days of Fast Therapy,"* well then, you can. If anyone you care for and who cares for you hears you say you can and watches you do it, they will feel the positive vibe. It's that simple. The difference is like night and day!

The mouthbody connection

While you may not see your esophagus, stomach, pancreas, intestines, liver, gallbladder, colon, rectum and anus in the same way you see your mouth, these organs are interconnected. All day long and at night when you're asleep (your liver is most active between 1-3 am), your visceral organs busily crosstalk with each other and with your brain and endocrine glands via messenger hormones and neurotransmitters that regulate digestion, absorption and elimination of food but also moods of depression/happiness, worry/joy, fear/faith and anger/acceptance.

Once you recognize the mouthbody connection as an aspect of the gutbrain connection, you naturally become more cautious, protective and strategic about what you put in your mouth, including food and drink but also pharmaceutical pills you're putting in your mouth every day and swallowing down without really thinking much about the risks and consequences for your visceral organs — especially when these synthetic chemical drugs were tested and approved for short-term use and weren't really designed for long-term use.

Regardless of what the pharmaceutical industry's marketing messaging says about managing chronic symptoms of physical and mental ill health by staying on your meds, be aware that the stress on your visceral organs may actually cause more depression, anxiety, OCD, ADD, agitation and mood swings over time. Because the root of the problem in your gut has not been addressed by chasing symptoms.

Honestly, it's a fantasy to think that popping a pill in your mouth can fix gutbrain imbalances and inflammation that are causing these imbalances in the first place. After a while, the stress on your liver and kidneys from metabolizing pharmaceutical drugs and eliminating the waste contributes to more imbalance and dysfunction. This is why studies are now showing the longer you stay on psychiatric drugs the greater your risk of both incontinence and dementia later in life. Dementia and incontinence are linked because of the gutbrain connection, and anyone who has visited a lockdown ward for the memory-impaired in a nursing home has seen firsthand the correlation between adult diapers, cognitive decline and overuse of pharmaceutical medications. The drugs don't address the root cause of chronic gut inflammation and loss of function, and over time the symptoms get worse.

Chronic negativity is a symptom

Just as there's a danger in putting too many things in your mouth that are unhealthy, toxic or even poisonous, there's also a danger in letting too much negativity come out of your mouth in your verbal speech, because negative feelings can somaticize and make you physically sick. And the reverse is also true. Pervasive negative thinking and speaking can be a symptom of bodymind illness and inflammation in your gutbrain. Either way you look at it, relentless pervasive negative thinking coming out of your mouth or the mouth of a loved one is actually an urgent call for help. If you know what I'm talking about because you suffer from chronic negativity yourself, take heart in knowing that every day of your fast brings relief because of the positive effects fasting has on the gutbrain connection. In the meantime, the exercises below will help you retrain your brain while your fast helps you heal your gut.

MOUTHPEACE EXERCISES

Exercise 1: Transform negative statements into positive ones that feel better

Review these examples of negative statements on the left transformed into positive ones on the right. Next, finish each negative statement in your own words, especially if it's something you hear yourself saying a lot, and then transform it into a statement that rings true but carries a positive charge.

Negative language	Positive language
You never...	
Ex. You never support me.	*I'd appreciate support right now.*
I never...	
Ex. I never get things done on time.	*I work at my own speed.*
I can't...	
Ex. I can't do this.	*I'm open to learning as I go.*
We can't...	
Ex. We can't do this anymore.	*We need better ways to communicate needs.*
I don't want to...	
Ex. I don't want to talk about it.	*This is difficult for me to talk about.*
Don't...	
Ex. Don't tell me what to do.	*Thank you for your concern.*

Identify a situation in which you heard yourself saying NO to a person in your life that ended on a sour note. Write down the negative statement you made. Whatever the situation was about, accept that when you said 'NO' you were trying to get a need met and were having difficulty. Identify what the need was that you were trying to get met.

Negative statement   **Need**

_____   _____

_____   _____

Next, articulate your need in positive language without using any negation words.

Need you wanted to get met   **Affirmative statement of need**

_____   _____

_____   _____

Exercise 2: Commit to purge negativity from your mouth during your fast

Go stand in front of a mirror, make eye contact with yourself, and say out loud, *"I commit to speak positive language today and every day of my fast."*

Negative words to avoid today and every day of your fast include *no, not, never, nothing, can't, won't, don't, couldn't, wouldn't, shouldn't, haven't, and nope — not happening.*

Do this exercise now and as a morning ritual every day of your fast. If you forget to look at yourself in the mirror and say, *"I commit to speak positive words today"* when you get up in the morning and go to the bathroom, put a post-it on the mirror to remind yourself to do it. For heady types who still believe the mind controls the body, trust me, thinking about doing something is different that physically doing it. You need to get the brainbody directly involved to change a somatic-emotional pattern. Every morning, stand in front of the mirror, look at yourself, and say the words out loud. Then go off into your day for the next ten days of your fast practicing positive language with a positive attitude and see how that works for you getting some needs met.

We say we "break" a habit for a reason. It's a process of becoming aware that you're doing something when before you were unaware, correcting yourself when you do it, and then over time just doing the new behavior and dropping the old one. So during your fast, as soon as you hear yourself making a negative statement, as soon as you become aware of it, or even feel yourself starting to go there, break your habitual pattern by slowing down and SAYING WHAT YOU DO WANT instead. Take the time to check in and feel what it is you really need, and then search for positive language to express your need, even if it takes a minute or two to feel, sense and think about what you really want to say. When you have the best words, then say it free of the burden and weight of negativity.

Practice makes perfect. Practice in earnest because your discipline is your freedom, but have fun with it, because it can be humorous and endearing. The other day my wife said to me, *"Your negative language doesn't stop me from seeing you as a positive person."* I had to laugh, because she was poking fun at me, but I took the cue and rephrased what I was trying to say in positive language. Our conversation went much better after that because, honestly, I only heard myself being negative when she pointed it out in her own witty way.

Exercise 3 for habitual naysayers: body test yourself when you say "NO"

If you experience yourself habitually saying NO and NOT before you even have time to sense your true feelings, you can end up negating the impulses, intuitions, desires and needs of those around you before you realize what you're doing. You can even negate your own feelings and needs in the blink of an eye.

"What's wrong?" someone asks. "Nothing, why?"

And just like that, you've shut down a conversation when it would have been more helpful to talk with emotional honesty about things that really matter when you can still do something about them. Maybe even ask for help or negotiate to get some needs met.

Words are fast, but the body is slower and needs more time. To break the habit of blurting out negative statements with a sharp tongue before you even have time to listen to the person talking to you to hear that person's needs, or listen to your own bodily sensations and feelings to know what you need, use this somatic technique to slow yourself down and give yourself more time to check in with yourself and others before you deliver a big package of negation to everyone.

Rather than say NO verbally, keep your mouth shut and shake your head NO in slow motion to body-test the negation to see if that's how you really feel.

Make the movement really slowly, turning your head several times left and right inch by inch, so you can sense how you feel in your body. Then check in to see how you feel. Does your NO feel authentic? Do you feel happy or sad as you shake your head? Calm or anxious? Empowered or disempowered? Do you feel angry or accepting? Do you feel needy or resourced?

Ask yourself where do I feel these negating feelings in my body? Touch that area of your body where you feel the NO. Place a listening hand there and listen to your embodied emotions.

Next nod your head YES up and down in slow motion to body-test an affirmation. Make it slow so you have time to feel your feelings. Do it several times.

Now check in with yourself. Does your YES feel authentic? Do you feel happy or sad as you nod your head YES? Calm or anxious? Empowered or disempowered? Do you feel angry or accepting? Do you feel needy or resourced?

If you feel some positive feelings when you say YES, place your hand on that part of your body. For example, let's say it's your son who is asking you to drive him somewhere when you are already stressed for time, so while you don't want to drive him you feel empathy for him wanting to get to this event he cares about because you love your son. You do want to help him, but you feel you don't have time. Place your hand on your heart where you feel love for your son (or your spouse, or friend, or whoever this person is to you.)

Now search for positive words to express how you really feel. Avoid negating words but express what you really feel and need.

With practice, you begin to easily find positive words to express the peaceful feeling you have when you say YES to what you *do* want rather than NO to what you don't want. Let those be the words that come out of your mouth, and then enjoy the peace that comes when you give the people in your life the opportunity to respond to what you do want rather than what you don't.

For example, in the case of the son who needs a ride, imagine saying *"I love that you want to go to your friend's birthday party, but I have a deadline tomorrow and I'm behind already, can you ask one of your friends if their mom could pick you up? And in the future, can you let me know in advance what you need so I can try to schedule for it?"* Talking in this way gets everyone's needs met with a positive vibe, even though the invitation to help is being declined.

DAY 2 ALL EARS

Chapter 5

All EARS —
Session Two

Day 2 of the fast

On Day 2 of your fast, you start fine tuning when you drink so that you are drinking *before* you feel hungry, such that your hunger goes into hibernation by Day 3. If you do this today, tomorrow you'll be *in the zone.* When your digestion shuts off, your energy is freed to fuel other functions including detoxification, elimination, cellular metabolism, immunity and hormone regulation. In the quietness of non-consumption, you can better hear the emotional crosstalk going on between your body and your brain. Listen carefully, you may be surprised at what you hear. It could be music to your ears, or a desperate plea for help, or the sound of distant footsteps coming. Whatever it is, let those with ears listen attentively and with curiosity to the bodymind connection setting the pulse of your embodied consciousness. The lesson and exercises in this session help you listen empathetically to parts of yourself and to people in your life in need of more love and care.

EMPATHETIC LISTENING

What you feel in your emotional bodymind when you're listening and how you respond affect you and the people you are relating to in a profound way. There is an art to listening. Being able to listen empathetically to someone else's experiences, feelings and needs, even when vastly different from your own, bonds you both in a field of connectedness that we all need to live well. Being listened to with empathy is healing, and being the empathetic listener for someone in need is also healing. It's healing for both people equally.

Our capacity to listen to each other and to feel empathy for each other enables us to bond with, communicate with, get in sync with, and learn quickly from each other. I don't need to burn my finger on a stove to learn that fire and heat can burn my skin and flesh. I can easily learn about being burned by empathizing with someone having that experience, even if that person was until that moment a stranger to me. Through empathy, I can learn about it almost as well by just hearing the story about what happened later, seeing the scar of the burn, and hearing about the distress and pain.

Imagine what it would be like if we couldn't do that. What if we all had to burn our fingers on a stove to learn that stoves can burn us. If it took us that long to learn something basic like that from each other, we humans would never have invented stoves in the first place. It's why in the classroom if we fail to establish empathy little learning takes place. The same is true in therapy. The same principle applies when we reach out to help people we care for and take care of at home, work and in our communities. And the same principle also applies when we listen to our own emotional, psychological and bodily needs when we practice daily self-care.

Empathy is different from sympathy

Sympathy comes easily with people to whom we are similar; we feel sympathy when we share someone else's experiences. Two angry people, two bullied people, two hurt people, two lonely people, two addicted people. Got it.

"I've been there," people say, giving a knowing look.

Sympathy explains why support groups like AA work so effectively, because it brings sympathetic people together to heal. But anyone who knows about AA knows that the rubber hits the pavement when you go back into your family to deal with family members who may have been soured, hurt and traumatized by the addiction, who because they weren't addicts can't sympathize the way a support group can.

Empathy is different. We empathize when we connect with someone who may be feeling emotions different from ours in response to experiences we haven't had. When we empathize, we feel what it would be like to **be** that other person going through those experiences. In essence, empathy is imagining another person in oneself. And vice versa, imaging oneself in another person. It's the ability to feel oneself walking in another person's shoes. And it comes with an attitude of good will toward the other person. When we say *"I feel you,"* that's empathy we're feeling.

Recovered addicts feel blessed when surrounded by people who feel empathy for them whether they can sympathize with them or not. But the truth is, all of us feel blessed by empathy. Especially if we're feeling unwell or out of balance or challenged in some way. We all naturally need empathy at times. It's part of how we heal.

Body metaphors

When you're *"all ears"* it means you're listening intently with an open heart and mind. It means you are eager to listen and that you're listening attentively and closely not only to what the other person is saying, but also to the feelings that person is experiencing when they talk. Often all that people in our life need from us is our listening empathetic ear. They don't need us to fix anything for them, but they do need to talk their feelings out and be heard with empathy and compassion. And so the phrase *"having his ear"* means having that person's attention and understanding. In this sense, *"to be heard"* means more than being audible, it means to be understood.

When someone *"turns a deaf ear to us"* it can be painful, because that person has closed their heart to us. No matter what we say with our words, the heart-to-heart connection we are seeking and needing isn't there. When a plea for help or support falls on deaf ears, it can feel devastating. *"How did it go? It didn't, she turned her ear to the wall,"* we say. Or we say *"it went in one ear and out the other."* And so it's a blessing when we have someone in our life who is willing and capable of *"lending an ear"* in times of need.

Anatomically, our ears are an organ for the perception of sound. But psychologically, they are more than just an organ of hearing; our ears are orifices by which we are touched and moved by our acoustic environment, a permeable boundary between our internal state of consciousness and sounds coming into us from the world.

> *Mother I hear you under my feet,*
> *Mother I hear your heart beat.*
> *Hey ya hey ya hey ya ho,*
> *Hey ya hey ya hey ya ho.*

While we can purposely turn our ears away from hearing something we don't want to hear, we can't really close our ears the way we can close our eyes. We hear things whether we want to hear them or not, whether it was *"music to our ears"* or *"poison to our ears."* Once we hear it, the vibration of it resonates within us, becoming part of our body memory, filling us with darkness and despair or light and hope.

Empathetic listening is a skill anyone can learn

There's an ancient adage that we have two ears and one mouth so that we can listen more than we talk. It's amazing what you can accomplish when you still your tongue and become all ears for a few minutes. The transfer of immense amounts of information can happen instantaneously when you stop talking and listen with ears connected to a feeling heart.

When we listen empathetically to people in our lives, we let the other people know we are actively listening to them and hearing them. By reflecting their words, their emotional affect and their body language back to them, we let them know they aren't alone in their vulnerability. We communicate that we feel for them and their situation, and that we care and are empathetically witnessing their pain, distress and needs. Reflection comforts and reassures a person who is in need of empathy.

Reflection also prevents us from projecting our own beliefs, desires and needs onto people in our lives. In this way, reflection provides safety for everyone. When we reflect, we mirror back what the other person is saying, emoting and doing. In contrast, when we project, we cast an image, belief, desire or feeling onto the other person as if they were a blank screen. Projections are external and can bear little or no relation to the person who is the recipient of them. They say more about the person projecting than the person who is the object of the projection.

Empathetic listening is comprised of rephrasing the content of what a person is saying so that they know they are being heard, and reflecting the emotions the person is expressing so that they know their feelings are being seen and felt. They know they are being understood on a deeper level. This is why empathetic listening is also called active listening. The listener is not listening in silence, rather the listener is actively engaged. In this way it feels like a conversation even though one person is doing most of the talking and the roles are very clear in this regard.

When listening empathetically to someone who needs to be heard and empathized with, we want to be mindful not only of our words but also our tone, pitch and volume. We want to use our voice like an instrument. The more you practice, the more you develop an ear for it. Be aware that many people have auditory sensitivity, and some are highly sensitive empaths. It takes self-awareness to use your voice like a musical instrument that sounds like music for tired ears rather than scratching nails on a chalkboard or a broken record.

Let's look at an example. If someone you care for comes to you with tears in their eyes, you can reflect that by saying, "I see tears welling up in your eyes." If you sense a cry coming up and the person is holding back, you might reflect "I see you holding your breath," and ask "do you feel like crying?" Then check in, let the person respond to you, to see if your sense of what's happening is accurate.

However, if you see tears welling up in a person's eyes and you jump ahead and say, "I see you're sad," that's actually a projection. Because while tears are very often an expression of sadness, those tears could also be tears of joy, or tears of frustration, or tears of physical or psychic pain. Rather than jump ahead and risk projecting, simply reflect what you're hearing, seeing and sensing, then check in and let the other person clarify and fill in the blanks. And then reflect their words and body language back to them to make sure you're following the body story.

Reflection increases empathy while projection can easily sound like judgments that can trigger reactivity and defensiveness that make it even harder to overcome differences between you and people in your life. Judgements and projections create separation and distance, so stick with reflection when you listen empathetically to those you care for and those in need. You'll find your conversations go much easier and your communication becomes much more effective. If you hear yourself projecting instead of reflecting, file those projections and come back to them later when you're focused on the work you do with yourself. They're full of juicy information about your own fears, judgments, desires, needs, attachments, thoughts, beliefs and habits.

Empathy is the foundation for emotional intelligence

In the heyday of Descartes' mind/body split, philosophers mistakenly thought that ethical thinking and behavior develop as a result of controlling and suppressing our emotions and body with our mind. But from a body psychology point of view, the opposite is true. Socially ethical behavior grows in the fertile soil of the emotion we call empathy. Without it, any of us can become lost in the proverbial wilderness. Today, we call it getting lost in the matrix. But whatever you call it, the important feature about it is the feeling so many people have of getting lost in it. Without empathy any of us can become socially alienated and feel hopelessly disconnected. And then it's difficult to maintain unity in shared values that are good for everyone involved. We close our hearts and stop listening.

However, when we practice empathetic listening, we exercise our ability to connect with, to know, to care for and to learn from the people around us — even people who are vastly different from us. Empathy bonds us and develops our internal sense of direction, belonging and purpose — including our moral sense of right and wrong. Because we only know what the right action is in any given situation when we feel empathy for the people around us who will be affected by our actions, when we feel enough love for them to care about them and care for them, and when we feel reverence for a collective existence larger than our own. We all need that to be well and to be at peace with each other.

Self-care for caretakers

If you're distracted when you reach out to care for someone, or feel anxious or agitated or sad, the other person will feel it immediately and your attempt to care for them may be short-circuited. Practice your own self-care before reaching out to help. Practice feeling empathy for yourself first to clear out some of your own somatic-emotional blockages that keep you from getting your needs met. In this way you'll have more resources to care for other people in your life.

There's a freedom in just listening to your own embodied emotions for a few precious minutes. It's enlightening to give yourself time to listen empathetically to all your parts, to become awake to these parts of yourself, to feel them, recognize their voice, hear them talking, and know them in a fully embodied way.

When fasting, you become much more aware of your visceral organs and their crosstalk with your limbic brain, somatosensory brain and cognitive brain. Listen to what your visceral organs need and want deep in your core. Because they can be the source of your bad moods and pains, your irritations and anger, even your fear and contempt. Stop talking at your body, telling it what to do, making demands on it, jamming it full of comfort food, taking risks with it, ignoring it, drowning it in drink or any other way you suppress your own bodily feelings. Because when cared for, our visceral organs can be the source of our good moods and pleasures, our patience and acceptance, and our joy and faith. Even our love.

Time to Listen

During fasting days, when someone you care for and who cares for you comes into your field of awareness and wants to express emotions or vent, settle in to be *all ears*. Give that person your whole attention. Forget about multi-tasking. That's a fantasy anyway, and even if you could multi-task, it would be ill advised for our purpose. For empathetic listening, we want to be 100% present and paying attention only to that person we are caring for.

Practice empathetic listening in the time you have to give — even if that's only a minute to touch an elbow or shoulder, make eye contact, and ask someone if they're okay before you tell them you have to take a phone call. Ask if you can come back to them later when you're done. And then make sure you follow up.

ALL EARS EXERCISES

Exercise 1: Listening with empathy to your parts

How many times have we heard of somebody suddenly getting a diagnosis seemingly without warning. *"They found it too late,"* we hear. This happens when people send early warning signs and pre-symptoms of chronic distress to the back closet of their psyche in an attempt to hide their situation because they feel so vulnerable. For preventive self-care, we want to bring these signals to the surface of our consciousness where we can touch them, feel them, talk about them and respond to them. Maybe even ask for help.

Locate a vulnerable part of yourself that is struggling and that you may have exiled out of self-protection. Reach out and touch this vulnerable, hidden-away part of yourself with a listening hand. Listen to this part of yourself with empathy and ask this vulnerable part of yourself what it needs to be well. Find simple words to reflect what you hear with your ears and what you feel in your hands. Maybe it's your heart, or your gut, kidneys, liver or colon. Maybe it's swollen, inflamed and stiff joints. Maybe it's your brain. Listen with an open heart and mind and accept that whatever symptoms of imbalance you suffer will resolve when your embodied needs are actually met. Listen to the crosstalk. Listen for the need being expressed. Identify that need.

Vulnerable part of you that is struggling

_____

_____

Need being expressed by that part of you

_____

_____

Exercise 2: Checking in with a hands-on body scan

Do a check-in with your visceral body. Lay an empathetic listening hand on your heart. Feel your own heartbeat. Is it fast, anxious and tense? Or calm, relaxed and peaceful? Do you feel loved or unloved? Loving or unloving? Your body knows the truth. What are you sensing in your heart right now? Say it out loud so you can hear it.

Next lay your listening hands on your stomach and your intestines and feel your body's truth there beneath your hands. Do you feel full, acidic, gassy, bloated, inflamed and foggy? Or do you feel empty, lean, satisfied, content and focused? Listen to your descending colon by laying a hand on your left lower abdomen where your descending colon is located. Is it empty and flat? Or do you feel feces there on its way to your rectum to be excreted? If so, how much feces? Is it a lot? Feel with your hands. Do an honest check-in and take the feedback. If you're chronically constipated, this part of you can become very distended, congested, inflamed and full of compacted feces that needs to be washed out and excreted.

Check-in with your kidneys that regulate your blood pressure and fluid levels through the secretion of the hormone vasopressin, and that regulate your stress response through the secretion of cortisol and adrenaline. Place your hands on your mid back on both sides of your spine just below your ribcage and hang out there while you listen empathetically to what your kidneys are saying to you. Are you constantly thirsty and dehydrated, anxious, fearful and irritated? Or do you feel satisfied when you drink, calm and full of faith that things will work out?

Touch your liver — the giver of life — tucked under the bottom of your right ribcage. It's a really large organ. Place your listening hands there and feel what's going on inside. If your liver is congested with toxic waste and dried up bile, and your gallbladder is full of calcified gallstones, well, you cannot be a happy person, can you? If your liver is unhappy in this way, you will find yourself full of bile, anger and resentment more than your friend who has a happy liver. And your heart won't be fully happy either, because your liver filters your blood and takes stress off your heart, and when it is functioning optimally, helps to regulate your blood sugar, blood pressure and blood cholesterol. True happiness in our embodiment is an expression of optimal self-regulation in all these organs. Whatever organ is calling out for attention and care, reach out and touch it. Locate it in your embodiment.

Identify the organ within you calling out for more care.

Organ in need:

_____

_____

Exercise 3: Empathetic listening with a partner

Sit down facing your partner. Get close enough that you can see each other's eyes and hear each other (even if whispering) and can comfortably reach out and touch your partner's knee, elbow or shoulder. Decide who is going to be practicing empathetic listening, and who is going to be the partner expressing emotions and feelings about something that has a vortex of energy around it. The partner who is going to share will say how they're feeling about something that has an emotional charge. The listening partner witnesses what comes out with their empathetic ears, rephrases using words, and reflects guttural expressions, emotional intonation and body language.

During this exercise, the listening partner maintains eye contact and the sharing partner follows their eyes wherever they want to move as they access the stinging memory that is carrying a charge. What that means is that the sharing partner will be coming in and out of eye contact, but whenever they look at the listening partner, that person is already looking back at them — rather than looking at their phone or glancing out the window! Listeners stay focused on your partner, whereas partners who are sharing allow yourself to follow the vortex of feeling that is challenging you wherever it goes.

In addition, the listening partner reaches out intuitively with empathetic listening touch in response to the emotional needs being expressed. Your body will know how to do this if you tune into your own gut intuition. Touch with guttural expression is the first language before words for newborns. We all understand this language. For example, if the sharing partner says, *"I felt so alone and frightened"* during a part of their body story, you can say, *"I'm here listening, I feel how much that frightened you"* while reaching out to lay your hand on your partner's shoulder or elbow to let them know that now, in the present moment, someone is there witnessing for them and caring for them. Your compassionate touch matches what your words are saying to communicate empathy in an integrated way that the brainbody understands.

If there is a lull in the talking, the partner who is empathetically listening can also get the body involved in the conversation by asking the sharing partner *"what are you feeling in your body? Where are you feeling it?"* Invite the person who is emoting to lay a listening hand on that part. Ask what this part would say if it had words, and then listen empathetically to the answer, reflecting the moods, feelings and words back to your partner.

Go for about 10-20 minutes, and then switch roles.

DAY 3
EYES WIDE OPEN

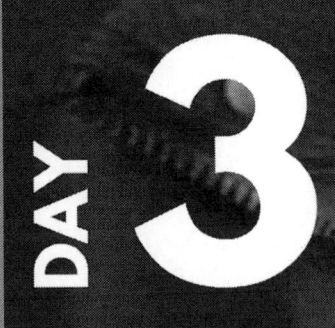

Chapter 6

EYES WIDE OPEN —
Session Three

Day 3 of the fast

On Day 3 of the fast, it can be enlightening to look into the toilet after a coffee enema and realize how much waste you've been carrying around inside of you. It's usually an eye-opening experience. Seeing is believing!

Eating constantly without taking a break to cleanse and restore your gut creates too much waste, especially if you've been eating nutrient-depleted foods that are high in refined sugar, flour and salt and contaminated with pesticides, herbicides, fungicides, additives and preservatives. The name of the game on Day 3 is to stay in the groove, stay on the path, and stay in the fast. Believe it or not, there's a lot more excrement in you that needs to come out, as you'll see for yourself a few days from now. The lesson and exercises in this session nudge you to open your eyes to the truth about your bodymind health and that of the people around you.

OBSERVING (YOUR) SELF

The state of consciousness you are in when your eyes are "wide open," and you can see the truth about yourself, liberates you from unnecessary pain and suffering. It's the ability to see what's right in front of your face when you look at yourself naked in a full body mirror. But it also includes what you see when you close your two visual eyes to look inward with your Observing Self at your own thoughts, feelings and behaviors.

The phrase *"eyes wide open"* describes the consciousness of the Observing Self that enables us to see without illusion or projection the truth staring us in the face. Being able to access the consciousness of the Observing Self whenever needed is liberating and empowering, for the simple reason that what you don't see and what you're not aware of about yourself can blindside you. You might find yourself saying *"I didn't see it coming"* when it was. Or *"it won't happen to me"* when it did. As a result, you end up losing precious time to turn yourself around with healthy changes when preventive self-care has the most impact.

However, once you become aware of your own mental, emotional and somatic behavior patterns, then you can change them. Once you can observe them for what they are, you can respond within your own embodiment to make adjustments and self-regulate. The sooner the better. Why wait until you're sick in mind, body and heart to adapt? Waiting too long to self-regulate is in and of itself maladaptive. Waiting can quickly turn into a long delay in seeing the truth about yourself and your current situation that would trigger healthy changes, until the opportunity to self-regulate passes, and imbalances become a chronic condition.

Loss of the ability to self-regulate is a characteristic shared by all chronic illnesses, and so we can identify it at the very root of the problem causing us so much suffering. There is the loss of the ability to self-regulate your own blood sugar levels in diabetes. Or the loss of the ability to self-regulate your own blood pressure in hypertension. Or loss of the ability to self-regulate the cholesterol in your blood in hypercholesterolemia. Or loss of the ability to self-regulate your own waste elimination in incontinence. It's the same for addiction, mental illness, cancer, obesity or autoimmune disorders. The characteristic they all share is loss of a core function of our embodied consciousness — the ability to regulate yourself, whether you're talking about your trigger-happy emotions and moods, your compulsive habitual behaviors, your consumption, your cellular metabolism, or your immunity.

Because of the legacy of the mind/body split in our society, many people today still mistakenly believe self-regulation is a mental process in which your mind manages your emotions and controls your body. However, this way of thinking is an illusion that feeds more ill health. Living in the illusion that our mind can regulate us or that smart technology can save us is the opposite of seeing clearly and being enlightened — which is what it feels like to "see" the bodymind connection without judgments or projections, to be aware of and awake to the reality of it, and to accept it for what it is.

Body metaphors

Body metaphors we use to describe the state of embodied consciousness when our eyes are wide open are either metaphors about being awake and waking up, or about seeing clearly and becoming enlightened. One famous example is the story of the Buddha being asked by someone, *"Are you a god or a man?"* To which the Buddha replied, *"I am awake."* Today we hear people say that someone *"had a wakeup call."* Johnny Nash evokes sunlight as a metaphor for seeing clearly in his classic pop hit *"I Can See Clearly Now."*

I can see clearly now, the rain is gone.
I can see all the obstacles in my way.
It's gonna be a bright, bright, bright sunshiny day.

It doesn't take long sitting quietly observing yourself before you realize that all your thoughts, moods and sensations are passing, and what remains over time is your Observing Self. It's like the sun in Nash's hit song. Every morning, no matter how dark the night or how long, the sun is still there shining down on you.

Self-acceptance

When you practice observing yourself with your eyes wide open, without judgment and without projection, you become aware of yourself as you are, and you get a fast pass to self-acceptance. Self-acceptance is accepting "what is" about yourself, including what you see when you look at yourself naked in a mirror, but also what you sense about yourself when you close your eyes to glance inward. If you can observe your own thoughts, feelings, beliefs, behaviors, attitudes and physical state of being, then those aspects of you that you can observe are not your Observing Self. Your Observing Self sees all of it and remains unchanging over time. So why identify with those aspects of yourself that are changing?

When experiencing pain and suffering in any given moment, it's even more painful to tell yourself that you are an unloved person, or unlovable person, or an angry person, or insecure person, or a sick person, or a depressed person, or an addict. Whatever it may be. Those thoughts are all judgments, and they feel heavy and disappointing. Soon enough you start thinking of yourself and your situation negatively.

However, it's easy to accept that you have a trauma trigger, or an addictive habit, or faulty logic, or an outdated belief system, or a sick gut, or an attachment to behaviors that are illness causing, or an unmet need. Maybe you even have symptoms that get you a medical diagnosis — a physical sign of your bodymind distress. It's critical to discern that the symptoms and diagnosis aren't you either. They are a part of you, indeed a very important part of you, but they aren't "You."

Many people who have healed from cancer insist on language that makes this distinction. They avoid saying "my cancer," and instead say "the tumor in my colon" or "the tumor in my breast," etc. The same principle applies to saying "my dementia." Think about it. When your goal is bodymind health and lifelong sustainable wellbeing, the right to "my dementia" as an identity, in other words, the right to be a memory-impaired person, sounds absurd on its face. It's unsane thinking any way you look at it. People suffering with dementia need our care, respect and acceptance, surely so, and also our compassion, but thinking that we all have the right to become cognitively impaired is unsafe. Dangerous even. If everyone thinks that way, imagine the implications. There won't be enough adult diapers for all of us, much less beds in nursing care facilities for the memory impaired.

There's a wonderful book written by a man who recovered from an Alzheimer's diagnosis entitled *Beating Alzheimer's.* The author Tom Warren tells how in the middle of utter discord and dysfunction in which he couldn't write a check anymore, or drive his car, or run the washing machine, somehow he miraculously still knew that he was more than the dementia diagnosis his doctor gave him. He refused to identify with the diagnosis.

His wife, a nurse, played a lead role in his healing journey — talk about family healing! They paired up to make fast and radical changes that produced effective results — starting with moving from a polluted metropolitan city to a coastal town by the seaside to get some fresh air and sunshine with lots of places to walk every day. His wife created a green home for them that was free of mold and neurotoxic volatile chemicals in the furniture, paint, flooring and cleaning products, and then set about nutrient-saturating him with organic whole foods including good fats like coconut oil and olive oil.

Very rigorously, she guided her husband through several liver detoxes. And at the same time found a holistic dentist who practiced systemic mouthbody dentistry to remove a mouthful of mercury amalgam dental fillings that were poisoning him. It took many trips to the dentist, but together they went through the process of getting this neurotoxic metal out of his mouth one quadrant at a time. It took discipline and patience, but in time Tom Warren experienced a total recovery, reversed his Alzheimer's diagnosis, and wrote a book to share his healing journey.

Think of his body story the next time it feels easier in the moment to do the same thing you've been doing and carry on with compensations you've developed that have become unconscious habits blocking you from getting your actual needs met. When it comes to preventive self-care, it's a game changer to see and accept what you've been doing about your bodymind health and how you've been living. It's faster to start your healing journey from here in the now — without judgments or projections and without pretending what's happening to you or someone you care for is something other than what it is.

Seeing with your 3rd eye

Whatever is beyond the purview of your Observing Self is subconscious. Sadly, there's little any of us can do about the consequences of our subconscious habits and beliefs other than suffer them. However, when we bring the unconscious into consciousness by observing our Self, we become more self-aware, and with self-awareness we develop more self-acceptance, self-love and self-knowledge — what we really need to take better care of ourselves and the people that we love and care for.

It can be helpful to close your two visual eyes to open your 3rd eye — the part of your Observing Self that sees and knows even with your two visual eyes closed. When we close our eyes in a state of waking consciousness, we naturally awaken our Observing Self that sees and knows in the dark without vision. What we call our 3rd eye is the area in our brain just inches behind our forehead where the hypothalamus, pineal gland and pituitary gland are situated, supported by the sphenoid bone that sits inside our skull above our palate and behind our visual eyes. It's shaped like a butterfly with wings spread out.

Our pineal gland hangs attached by a short stalk to a fluid-filled ventricle in the midline of our brain. This area of our bodymind functions like a switchboard where all our systems connect in a fast freeway for crosstalking messenger hormones. Our 3rd eye *is* our bodymind connection. At the very seat of self-regulation, the hypothalamus receives messages from our body via neurohormones that trigger our pineal gland to secrete hormones that activate our pituitary gland located just below it. Called the master gland, the pituitary in turn secretes messenger hormones used around our bodymind to regulate multiple functions necessary to sustain good health, including stable moods, sleep, fertility and metabolism.

How our 3rd eye "sees" has been described as lucid dreaming and psychic visions. It is the source of insights and foresight, creative epiphanies and paradigm shifts. It's the seat of self-knowledge, wisdom, social ethics and morality — your sense of what's right or wrong. And it's your internal sense about how to find your way home when you're tossed at sea or lost in a forest or spinning in the matrix. To see with your 3rd eye open is the very definition of being enlightened. Our 3rd eye is light sensitive. It's the part of us that orients the crown of our skull to point up toward the sun and guides us to stand up vertically on two legs to walk the Earth. It is the visionary part of our embodied consciousness — the part of us that sees the truth of what is and also the possibility of what could be.

Ayurveda, Chinese medicine, natural medicine and tribal shamanic medicine all use prevention-oriented bodymind practices that have sustained people's health for thousands of years. All of them have practices to develop the Observing Self — whether it's meditation, yoga, prayer, chanting, Ayahuasca ceremonies, sitting in a pitch-black sweat lodge, or plunging in an ice-cold bath — all of which will put any of us in a deep meditative state within minutes if not seconds.

These bodymind practices work by evoking a resting state of connectivity, as neuroscientists call this specific state of brainbody connectivity that happens when we sit quietly doing nothing. When you evoke this state, you quickly recognize that something has changed, and that something that changed is your inner state of embodied consciousness. You become more calm, less reactive, less stressed and more detached, and at the same time more aware and more "connected." You may experience sudden insights, intuitions, visions and waking dream states. The physical effects can be measured in your heart rate, blood pressure and hormone levels, including cortisol (stress) and insulin (blood sugar). It is a state very different from sleeping because you're restful but awake. And in this calm awakened state doing nothing and free of the distraction of any specific task, your bodymind connections pulse with energy and consciousness. As long as you are busy doing something, you cannot access this state of consciousness and connectivity.

If you feel worried or anxious when you observe yourself, reassure your worried mind that nutritional wet fasting nurtures your capacity to be in a state of detached awareness. With every day that goes by on your fast, your brain and nerves become more hydrated and nourished rather than starved and dehydrated, and your physical body detoxifies and eliminates neurotoxins such as pesticides, petroleum chemicals, plastics, polychlorinated biphenyls (PCBs), and heavy metals like lead, arsenic and mercury. Take heart knowing that 10 days of nutritional wet fasting provides your brainbody what it really needs to "wake up." Expect more and more 3rd eye activity as you go deeper into your 10-day fast.

EYES WIDE OPEN EXERCISES

Exercise 1: Tapping to awaken your 3rd eye

This exercise is a fast way to turn down the stress and wake up your 3rd eye (pineal, pituitary and hypothalamus) by tapping on your skull. Your two visual eyes will naturally want to close for this, and you will find some relief for eye strain.

Start by tapping your forehead between your eyebrows and slightly above them with the fingertips of your index and middle finger. Tap gently and rhythmically for about 30 seconds, while gently pressing the tip of your tongue into the ridge of your upper palate.

Next tap your crown chakra at the very top of your skull with the fingertips of all five fingers including your thumb. Tap gently and rhythmically for about 30 seconds, while gently pressing the tip of your tongue into the ridge of your upper palate.

Cycle through 3 sets of tapping for 30 seconds on your 3rd eye point followed by tapping for 30 seconds on your crown point.

When you finish, give yourself a minute to feel and sense what's going on inside your skull. What did you feel in your fingertips when you tapped? What did you feel in your skull bones when you tapped? What did you feel in your upper palate? Did you feel the vibration inside your brain? And more specifically, in your hypothalamus, pineal gland and pituitary gland? Could you feel the inside of your skull as well as the outside when you tapped? What do you feel now in your 3rd eye? Is it cold or hot? Is it tender or sore? Did any feelings or visuals come up for you?

Exercise 2: Mirror exercise to develop self-acceptance

Spending time with your Observing Self increases self-awareness and teaches self-acceptance and self-love — two drivers for effective self-care. Self-awareness is naturally a game-changer for relationships too. "Know thyself" is a responsibility we all share before we relate to others. Self-awareness comes in handy when someone who cares for you asks you why you don't take better care of yourself.

Write the affirmations below on a piece of paper and tape it to your bathroom mirror.

I love you.
I respect you.
I accept you.
I am.

During fasting days, whenever you go to the bathroom and see your paper with affirmations, pause for a moment to look in the mirror and say these healing statements to yourself. When you bathe or shower, take a minute to look at yourself naked in the mirror, and say the words to yourself.

As you practice self-acceptance without judgment during your fasting days, observe how you respond to the affirmations and how your response changes over time.

Exercise 3: Discerning observations from judgments

The part of you that makes judgments is different from your Observing Self. Your Observing Self can observe your own judgments, even as another part of you is making them. Think of a time when you realized your judgment about someone's motivations were off. Or a time you thought something was true that turned out to be false. The part of you that was able to observe yourself making that mistake is your Observing Self.

Look at these examples of judgments that have been downgraded into simple observations. Notice the change in emotional tenor and mood that accompanies the change in language when you go from judgments and evaluations to neutral observations.

Judgment	Observation
You were a jerk!	*I saw you turn red in the face and storm out.*
You insulted me!	*You said I'm selfish.*
You're manipulating me.	*I hear you want me to agree with you.*
It's your fault.	*I hear myself blaming you.*
You're a worry wart.	*I can hear you're worried.*

Think of a judgment you made about someone you care for. It could be recently or long ago. Write down your judgment, then downgrade that judgment into a neutral observation.

Judgment I made: *Neutral observation:*

_____   _____

_____   _____

Think of a judgment you made recently or long ago about yourself. Write down that self-judgment and then change it into a neutral observation.

Self-judgment I made: *Neutral observation:*

_____   _____

_____   _____

Exercise 4: 20-minute meditation

Daily morning meditations develop your Observing Self. You can optimize your Fast Therapy by sitting for a 20-minute morning meditation during fasting days. But keep in mind that morning meditations are just practice for when it matters most — which is when the proverbial shit hits the fan in your life. With a little practice, you learn that you can stop whatever you're doing to meditate and get the same results even if it's on a public bench in the middle of a busy shopping center or surrounded by chaotic noises at home or work. Eventually, if you meditate long enough, you learn you can keep your 3rd eye open and active when your two visual eyes are open too.

Sit down with comfortable back support, close your eyes, and focus your attention for a few minutes on your breath passing in and out of your nostrils. Narrow your attention down to just your nasal breathing passing in and out of your nose. As your breathing slows and deepens, your nervous system begins to unstress and you can feel yourself drop down into a deeper state of relaxation as your brain wave frequency slows from faster beta to slower alpha and theta.

After a few minutes, you will notice it becomes easier to sense and feel your inner state of being as your attention shifts from external perceptions to internal interoception. Observe any thoughts flitting by or emotions rising up without feeling like you have to do anything about them or react to them in any way. But if you do (and everyone knows it happens) and you find yourself sucked into a vortex of memories, feelings and sensations, breathe into them and allow yourself to feel whatever is happening in your body. Just observe what's happening without feeling you have to do anything about it.

Continue to meditate for about 20 minutes. No need for an alarm or anything external like that. About 20 minutes and you'll know when you're done. If you go longer, hey, it happens. If you go shorter, whose counting? If you fall asleep it means you're exhausted and need to sleep because you're starved for REM. So let yourself sleep and try meditating again when you're rested.

When you finish your meditation, give yourself a couple minutes before you open your eyes to integrate what you've experienced as you shift into your waking state consciousness with your eyes open. Over time, as you practice your meditation consistently, you develop more detachment, less reactivity and more insight.

DAY 4 SKIN DEEP

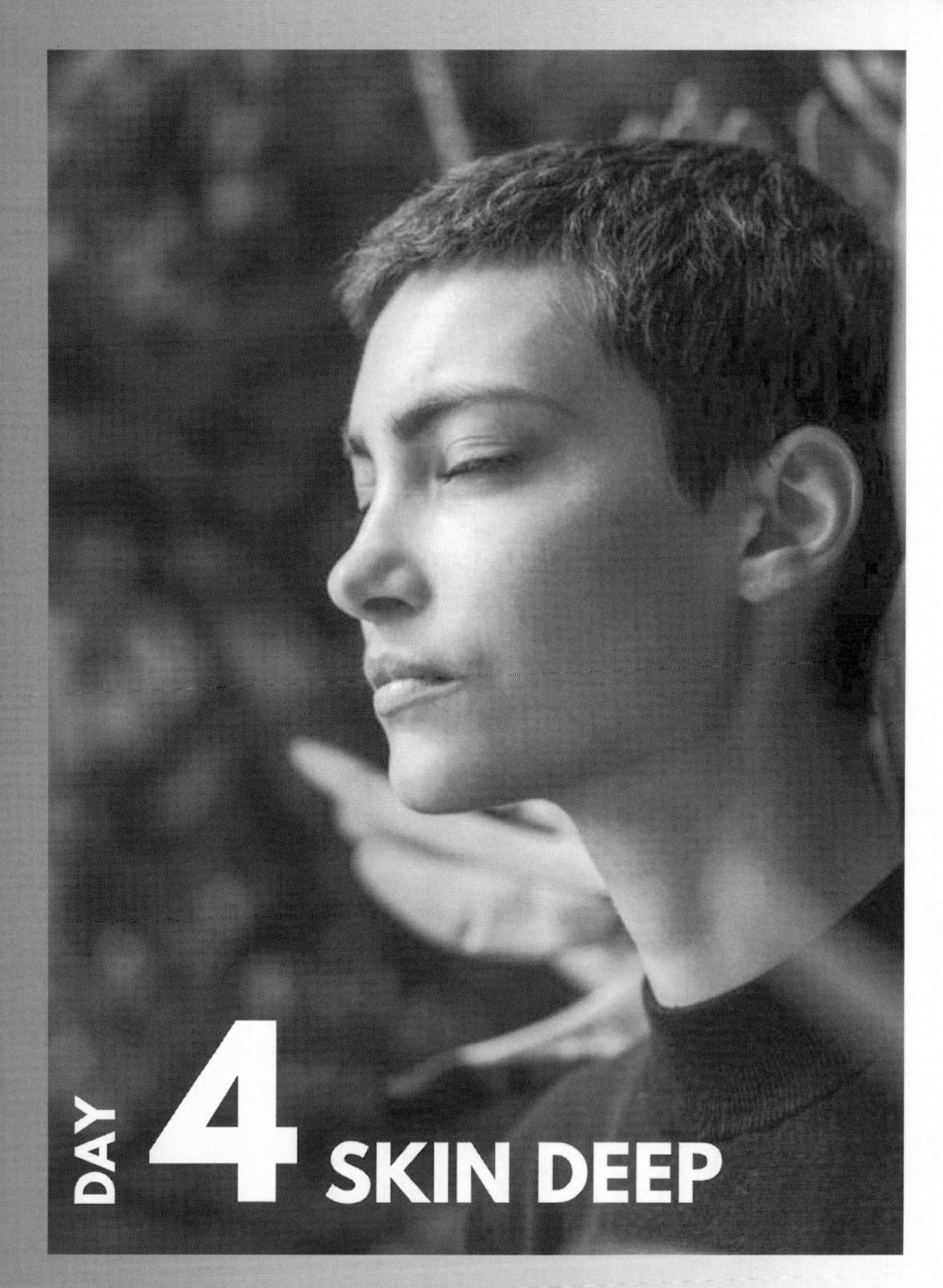

Chapter 7

SKIN DEEP —
Session Four

Day 4 of the fast

After three full days of drinking your daily drinks and eliminating acidic waste faster, you are becoming more alkaline. And the more alkaline you become within, the more the gradient effect kicks in, and the more acidic waste is pushed out from your cells to be purged. The River of Life you've created to wash yourself clean from within is gushing by Day 4, flushing out the excrement of the past and feeding bioavailable nutrients to your visceral organs.

Your attention will naturally be drawn to what's going on inside your visceral body, deep beneath the surface of your skin. Go there. Today is an opportune time to dive beneath the surface to get a reality check on your core health. Same goes for the people you care for. Take a look to see what is right there in front of you just beneath the skin. If you see something is out of balance, reach out and touch it. Start the conversation. Sometimes we all need that reality check. The lesson and exercises in this session help you dive deep beneath cover stories that block you and the people you love from talking about what matters most when it comes to your bodymind health. Dive in.

COVER STORIES

Have you ever felt like you were listening to an old recording of worn-out excuses and explanations when you ask someone about their health? Or maybe you are the one to hit the play button when someone asks, "How are you?" As soon as the conversation starts to deepen, it feels like someone is suddenly running a recording on auto-play. That's a cover story, and it can keep you and the people you love from taking better care when it matters most.

"He has an iron stomach; he can eat anything" was a cover story surrounding someone who died of stomach cancer. He believed his own cover story, and everyone who knew him participated in it. They thought that if they fed him treats, or fed him more, it would make him happier.

Cover stories are often repeated out of habit, until they sound familiar. Families and friends share them and circulate them. They come wrapped with an invitation for everyone who hears them to be complacent and go along, staying on the surface and not diving deeper. They can feel like an unspoken agreement. *"Let's not talk about it,"* cover stories say. They cut deeper conversations short or shut them down altogether. They're conversation closers.

"Are you sure you want a pastrami sandwich for lunch again? Last time you ate one you had horrible indigestion."

"I'm fine, don't worry about me, I have an iron stomach."

"Oh, okay then, I know a great Italian market where we can get a cherry soda and a pastrami. My treat!"

Just like that, a window of opportunity to get to the truth of ill health opened and closed. Life moved on, and the conversation about what mattered most never happened, until a time came when it was too late to either ask for help or reach out a helping hand. Too late is a very sad time, and many wonder if our species on this planet has hit our "end times." All of us together. Is it too late for us to turn our health around? Is it too late for you, or for me? And for the people we love? There's only one way to find out, because staying of the surface obsessed with appearances in social media posts is part of how we got here where we are, a time when so many people are falling ill.

The next time someone says "*I'm fine*" when they're not, slow down. Accept that the story is just beginning. Make eye contact and gather your parts to dive deeper than the skin of the story to discover the truth that the body is telling. It might be a story of pain and discomfort and the emotions that go with pain and discomfort. Sadness and anxiety. Grief and regret. Fear. Maybe it's your fear, maybe it's your grief. Ask yourself, are you willing to dive deep to get to the bottom of it?

Body metaphors

The phrase *"skin deep"* implies staying on the surface, minimizing and concealing until the inevitable moment of revelation when the body story pushes through and ruptures a cover story with its deeper truth. Suddenly "I'm fine" turns out to be "I'm not fine at all." People intuitively understand that when something is *"skin deep"* it's just a surface appearance, and one would be foolish to trust it.

Common body metaphors for cover stories refer to superficiality. *"Their loyalty was only skin deep,"* we say, meaning the loyalty was merely the appearance of loyalty on the surface. Or we say, *"her beauty is only skin deep"* when what's beneath the surface is less than beautiful, even if what you see on Instagram is picture-perfect. Vice versa, we say someone is being *"totally transparent"* when they forego appearance and pretense for brutal honesty.

The ability to see through cover stories to get to the truth that the bodymind is telling is a skill all of us can develop. We need this skill when it comes to caring for our bodymind health and the health of people we love. Especially when cover stories are everywhere in the media, and cover stories mislead us into doing nothing when something could have been done.

For example, there's a pervasive cover story that circulates through the news cycle that pretends there's little direct connection between our high cancer rate in the U.S. and environmental contamination with ionizing radiation from nuclear technology, when in fact there is a clear connection. But let's not talk about it, because if we don't talk about it, it's not real, right? And if it's not real, then we can plan a nuclear renaissance and plow forward into our nuclear future, seemingly unaware of the implications for all life on the planet.

However, if you're willing to touch the truth and be touched by it — including symptoms of ill health just below the surface of what can be talked about in a cover story — you'll naturally be able to take better care of yourself and the people you care for. Because you'll be able to stop pretending everything's fine and respond in an adaptive way to what is.

Touching the visceral body story

It takes courage and compassion to look symptoms of chronic bodymind illness in the face and talk about them, especially when 52% of Americans already have one or more chronic condition, including mental health conditions. It takes heart to be willing to sense the deeper body story beneath the surface, touch it and listen to it, including what it says about how we may have made ourselves ill, personally and collectively. And about what we need to do to turn ourselves around. That deeper story is told in the body, where sensations and feelings of discomfort, pain and loss of function are experienced and remembered in the visceral organs, loaded with the impulse to discharge their story when triggered. When you go deep, it gets deep fast. Be willing to go there to look the truth in the face. Reach out and touch the part of you that is hiding behind a cover story about your health.

Let's do it together right now. Reach out and touch your liver with your empathetic listening hands. I'm touching mine right now, feeling it beneath my skin. It's a large organ tucked under the right rib cage. Bring your awareness to what you are sensing internally there. People are so obsessed with their face these days, and forget to care for their liver, the giver of Life. Breathe in and out of your nose quietly while you listen and hold your liver in your hands. Cradle your liver and listen to it. What story is this organ telling about the current state of your wellbeing? About the choices you've made and the life you've lived? Feel your liver's story. Is it swollen, inflamed and congested? Painful even to the touch? Does it feel enlarged and fatty? Does it feel angry and hardened with dried-up bile and calcified gallstones in its gallbladder? Or is it happy and hydrated and loving your life? Ask your liver what it would say if it had words.

Work around your body this way, touching and talking to all your parts, listening and deepening the conversation we could all be having with ourselves and each other. If you have a bloated and inflamed belly, lay your hands on your belly and start a conversation with your belly's story, how it came to be the way it is today. Hold your intestines and colon in your hands and listen to what these organs are telling you. Whatever part of you is calling out for care, touch it and talk to it. Search for feelings words that are authentic to say the things that might be hard to speak. And at every twist and turn in the journey, whenever there's an invitation to stay on the surface and keep it superficial, ask a deepening question to follow the body story down to the bottom of it. Let your relationship with yourself be visceral, not just visual. Look at what's right in front of your face just beneath the skin. And find the words to talk about it.

Getting to the bottom of it

While it may feel easier in the moment to stay on the surface and go along with a cover story, deep healing only happens from the bottom up. When a wound heals on the surface but not underneath, an abscess can form. The wound will have to open again and again to heal completely. Healing from the bottom up is the fastest way, even though it takes more time than putting a band-aid on the superficial skin of the situation, and then dealing with it again later when it comes back up to the surface with more intensity.

For these reasons, during fasting days, kindly decline to go along with a cover story when you hear one. When someone you care for looks like they could use a helping hand and an empathetic ear, dive deep with them rather than stay in the shallows. Be curious and courageous. Ask the questions that matter most to keep the conversation going. Get to the bottom of it. Whatever it is. Do the same for yourself when you hear yourself telling a cover story to someone who cares for you who is reaching out wanting to help.

SKIN DEEP EXERCISES

Exercise 1: Asking deepening questions

Look at the different types of common cover stories below on the left with deepening questions on the right. I give you two examples. You take it from there and come up with some questions in response to the remaining prompts. If you feel you are getting lost in the woods, imagine what the emotional and physical needs are and deepen in that direction.

Cover story	Deepening question
20 reasons. Ex. I lost my wallet again; I was in a rush. Last week I was distracted by my son.	*You've been losing a lot of things lately, are you concerned about your memory?*
Minimizing. Ex. Who needs a life partner, I have enough troubles of my own.	*How does that work for you when you need intimacy?*
Pushing through. Ex. I'm always exhausted after lunch, I need another coffee.	
The temporary fix. Ex. My hair is falling out, I'll try a new shampoo.	
The brush off. Ex. I'm fine. Don't worry about me.	

Exercise 2: Uncovering your cover story

Learning to ask deepening questions is actually easier than it may at first feel. Honestly, just saying *"tell me more"* and redirecting the conversation back to emotions and sensations in the body when you don't know what to say is a simple skill anyone can master. It sounds like this, *"Tell me more about your indigestion Richard, last time we had lunch you were really in pain and looked pale, and I noticed you've been taking a lot of Pepto Bismal with your meals. Your belly is so distended. What's going on?"* All it takes is a willingness to dive deeper beneath the surface to get to the visceral body story beneath the cover story. Be gentle but persistent, because only the truth will set any of us free.

Keeping that in mind, bring your attention to a cover story you've heard yourself tell recently about your bodymind health and wellbeing, including your physical, emotional, mental and spiritual health. Sit down with your Observing Self and your empathetic ears to listen to the deeper truth beneath your cover story.

Start by bringing your attention to the part of you that told the cover story. Put a listening hand there on that part of you. Was it your manager, trying to manage the situation? Or was it your frightened exiled child who grew up neglecting yourself and hiding your needs in the shadows? Was it your firefighter putting out a fire? Where in your body does this part of you live? Place a listening hand there. Ask this part of you what it needs to let go of telling cover stories.

Next, name any chronic signals being suppressed by that cover story you told recently. Is it stomachaches, kidney pain, gallbladder pain, arthritic joints in your hand? Is it your brain? Is it an addiction to putting something in your mouth or sinuses or smoking it into your lungs? Identify where in your visceral body the issue is and place a listening hand on the visceral organ or organs involved. Listen to the body story. Ask that part of you a question that deepens the conversation. See if you can get to the bottom of any signals that are coming to the surface to express. Ask those signals your deepening question and be patient. Wait for the end of the story.

DAY 5 IN TOUCH

Chapter 8

IN TOUCH —
Session Five

Day 5 of the fast

By Day 5 of a 10-day fast, emotions are on the move as your visceral organs detox acidic waste to be eliminated from your body. Today is a good day to test your morning pH to see if you're in the ideal range yet, around 7.4 pH. The amount of waste coming out of you might surprise you. Remember to do your coffee enema to stay in the detox flow. You might find yourself getting emotional around Day 5 as your bodymind detoxes feelings from different organs, pushing them to the surface to release. Today's lesson and exercises help you get in touch with those feelings and the organs that regulate them. Today is a good day to get to know yourself better in your emotional body. What makes you tick. Obsess. Get anxious, angry or depressed. You'll be using your hands in the exercises to reach out to touch parts of yourself that are talking that you may have been forgetting to listen to.

GETTING IN TOUCH WITH YOUR EMOTIONS

Being human is being vulnerable. We are born vulnerable, and we die vulnerable. When we're sick, we're vulnerable. When we lose a loved one, our home, or our health, we're vulnerable. Trying to hide our vulnerability is a waste of precious time. Why fake it? Whatever it is that's out of balance — touch it, feel it, look it in the face, and talk about it with emotional honesty to heal it faster.

So many of us live in societies that have forsaken the emotions and exalted the rational cognitive mind. We were told this way was more civilized. We were told that smart technology is better than our human technology at everything from conceiving and birthing babies to fighting off a cold.

Yet look around. Here in the United States, Americans have the highest chronic illness rates, including mental illnesses, of comparable industrialized nations around the world, even though we spend more money on health care. Higher heart disease rates. Higher cancer rates. Higher diabetes rates. Higher rates of kidney disease, arthritis and dementia. According to "Quality of Health Care System Stats" from Nation Master's 2023 report, the U.S. spent twice as much as France on health care for nowhere near the efficacy. France ranked #1 in skill and competence of medical staff, ranked #3 in cost, and ranked #3 in overall quality of health care system. In comparison, after spending twice as much money as France on healthcare, the U.S. ranked #16 in skill of medical staff, #23 in cost, and #41 in overall quality of care. Perhaps what Americans are missing is emotional honesty about our chronic poor healthcare. Are we just out of touch?

Body metaphors

Body metaphors for the connection between your body, mind and emotions often have to do with *"being in touch"* or being *"out of touch."* We say someone is *"in touch with their feelings"* when they are being emotionally honest, or we say we were *"touched"* by their expressions of empathy and compassion. When we talk that way, we are acknowledging that we feel our emotions in a very physical way. We are touched by our feelings. We are moved by them. They affect us. And we can be in touch or out of touch with these feelings to greater or lesser degrees mentally, somatically and psychologically.

During fasting days, we want to be in touch with our emotions and the emotions of others as much as possible. We want to explore our feelings, get to know them and understand them. Be your own empathetic witness to your feelings. If you feel depressed or anxious or angry or irritable, and you don't like what you're feeling, it helps to own those feelings and take responsibility for them by understanding where they're coming from. When you can do that consistently for yourself, it's easier to be in touch with the feelings of people around you.

The scale of the emotions

Manfred Clynes, who developed the first machine to measure emotions, used the word "sentic" to denote the language of the emotions as distinct from the cognitive language of semantics and the physical language of somatics. To be healthy, we need all three languages to express in an integrated way. When what we feel and what we say and what we do are all integrated, it becomes so much easier for people to understand us and for us to get our needs met.

All our emotions are adaptive in certain situations — even rage and fear. If your house is burning down, fear is the most appropriate emotional response and can motivate you to flee for your life. Likewise, anger is a healthy emotional response to injustice. But getting stuck in one emotion like chronic anxiety or chronic anger or chronic depression is unhealthy. It blocks you from feeling the full range of your emotions which naturally express up and down the scale of emotions in response to events happening in your life. Healthy emotional expression uses the whole emotional scale, including the high notes.

Because of the way our embodied emotions express on a scale, the remedy for too much of a negative, heavy emotion is more of the opposite feeling in our lives. For example, too much fear is balanced by more faith. Too much anger is relieved by more acceptance. And the remedy for too much grief is more gratitude.

A friend of mine once shared that she was flying to attend the funeral of the husband of a friend of hers who died quietly of heart failure in their bed one night. He was only in his 40s. When she returned from her trip, I asked her how her friend was at the memorial service. She reported that this friend was doing remarkably well and was an inspiration to everyone at the service. Her friend expressed that she was grateful for all the years she had with her husband before his passing. They both knew he had heart problems that might bring his end sooner than most. And so they lived their life as if each day might be their last together. Now, though he was gone, she had two children in whom she could see his spirit living on. Her gratitude was greater than her grief, and people at the memorial service could feel that. It gave everyone there the heart to go on even though everyone was grieving.

Sensory awareness of emotions

If you're so used to disconnecting from your feelings, dissociating, shutting down your emotions or pleasing other people that you can't remember what emotional honesty feels like, take a deep breath. Close your eyes. Tune into your bodily sensations. Feelings are different than thoughts because you *feel* them in your body.

For this reason, long-winded talk in which you string together long sentences when you try to say how you *feel* is a sign that your "manager," your cognitive mind, has stepped in to take over and manage your emotions. When that happens, go back to silent nasal breathing, 4-count in and 4-count out, and just allow yourself to feel what's going on inside. Following your breath will help you shift your attention from racing thoughts or controlling thoughts back to your felt senses and embodied emotions.

Check in with your body. What are you feeling in your heart? Use an empathetic listening hand to touch your heart. What are you feeling in your gut? Use an empathetic listening hand to touch your belly. Maybe it's your brain. Or maybe it's your eyes. Maybe it's your exhausted adrenal glands or thirsty dried-up thyroid asking for iodine, selenium and living water. Reach out and touch that part of you. Be honest about what you're feeling in your body. Listen empathetically.

When you've listened quietly for a few minutes (remember the mind is fast whereas the body is slow, so give yourself time), ask that part of you that you are touching what it would say if it had words. Listen to what these parts of you tell you in the language of the emotional body. Trust that whatever it is that needs healing, the fastest way to take care of it is to touch it, feel it, and talk about it with emotional honesty. It takes practice being connected to your emotions if you are unaccustomed to doing so. Be willing to practice.

Developing emotional intelligence

Emotional intelligence is the ability to perceive, understand and communicate emotions. In the age of bullying and shooting sprees in schools, I think we can all recognize that cognitive intelligence without emotional intelligence is a recipe for disaster.

Being *dis*honest about our emotions is a way of suppressing them, and all we end up doing by suppressing our emotions is confusing ourselves and the people relating to us, because dishonesty makes it harder to be understood. Emotional dishonesty turns communication into a cognitive maze that's easy to get lost in. It makes self-care and being cared for by others unnecessarily difficult. And over time, emotional dishonesty can make us physically sick by blocking the release of pent-up emotions that need to discharge to come to completion.

As you develop your ability to be in touch with your emotions and to be emotionally honest about what you feel, you develop more emotional integrity. Emotional integrity is your personal capacity to feel and act on your authentic emotions that remains constant even under stress. If you have emotional integrity when you express thoughts, words and actions in your life, you express who you really are, what you really care about, and what you really need to be happy and whole. You also discover how the people in your life honestly feel about you when you are being authentic to your own feelings.

GETTING IN TOUCH EXERCISES

Exercise 1: Cycling through the scale of emotions

Complete each sentence below in your own words to help you cycle through the scale of emotions. Get in touch with each feeling as you do this exercise by referencing body memories to help you access the sensory feeling of each emotion. Lay a listening hand on where in your body you feel each emotion. Observe which emotions are familiar to you and which are unfamiliar. Identify where on the emotional scale you spend most of your time. After you complete the exercise, find someone to share your results with and discuss any insights that came up for you.

Fear (kidneys)	**Faith**
I'm afraid of...	*I have faith in...*
Control (colon)	**Detachment**
I obsess over...	*I feel detached about...*
Anger (liver)	**Acceptance**
I'm angry about...	*I accept that...*

Grief (lungs)	**Gratitude**
I feel grief over...	*I feel gratitude for...*
Regret (pancreas)	**Joy**
I regret...	*I feel joy over...*
Greed (stomach)	**Satisfaction**
I want more of...	*I'm satisfied with...*
Depression (intestines)	**Happiness**
I'm unhappy because...	*I'm happy about...*
Loneliness (heart)	**Love**
I feel disconnected from...	*I feel connection with...*

Exercise 2: Touching your emotional body

Think of a situation in your life in which you felt an intense negative emotion. Maybe you felt sad. Maybe you felt angry. Maybe you felt anxious or afraid. Maybe you felt grief. Maybe you felt heartache. Maybe you were worried sick. Connect the feeling you felt to the organ that regulates it by placing a listening hand on that organ. For example, if you felt angry touch your liver. If you felt anxious or fearful touch your kidneys. If you felt lonely or heartbroken touch your heart. Feel for any inflammation, congestion or discomfort in that part of you. Ask that part what it would say if it had words. Listen empathetically to that part of your emotional bodymind.

What the organ, gland or part of you is saying:

_____

_____

Exercise 3: Identifying emotional needs

Review these examples of emotions and the needs they express. Then complete each sentence in your own words and be emotionally honest. Identify the unmet need driving each emotion.

Emotion	Need
I'm afraid of...	**I need...**
Ex. being single forever.	*commitment.*
I'm angry that...	**I need...**
Ex. you snapped at me in front of guests.	*respect.*
I resent...	**I need...**
Ex. helping you when later you ignore me.	*reciprocity.*
I'm depressed because...	**I need...**
Ex. we have the same fight over and over.	*more happiness.*
I worry that...	**I need...**
Ex. I'll run out of time.	*stress relief.*

DAY 6 GUT FEELINGS

Chapter 9

GUT FEELINGS —
Session Six

Day 6 of the fast

By Day 6 you've flushed pounds of fecal waste from your gastrointestinal tract, starved parasitic yeast if you had an overgrowth, and nourished your intestinal mucosal lining with a nutrient-rich River of Life long enough to feed beneficial gut bacteria. Some of those beneficial bacteria help make messenger neurohormones for the gut-brain axis that connects your central and enteric nervous systems. For example, 90% of your serotonin, the happy hormone, is made in your gut.

It's common to feel flushes of feel-good moods in the middle of a 10-day fast. After a coffee enema pushes even more waste from your liver, you might even feel high. The effect on your central nervous system of changes in your gut microbiome and your gut's inflammatory immune response is fast. Especially when metabolic waste is coming out of your liver and colon more than food waste because you haven't eaten food in 6 days. Fasting instigates a deep cellular cleansing; as you become more alkaline, your organs and glands release their acidic waste and start to function more effectively.

The lesson and exercises in this session help you facilitate this release so you can hear your gut feelings easier. Move today, take a walk, keep it flowing. Keep drinking.

Some people, however, may feel crappy on Day 6. If you came into your fast with sugar-cravings from habitually eating sugar and carbs or drinking sugar in the form of sodas or alcohol, you may have an overgrowth of yeast in your intestines that are starting to die-off. Search "candida yeast in toilet" on Google Images and you'll see it if you haven't seen it already. Stalks of yeast buds that are stringy and yellowish brownish. The die-off of candida is neurotoxic and can make you feel foggy, tired, irritable and toxic. Remember to take a charcoal binder today and do a coffee enema even if you feel lethargic.

If you have an overgrowth of yeast in your belly, you might also want to do a Candida yeast cleanse with xylitol today to help yourself out. Obviously, the best time to cleanse yeast from your body is when your intestines are empty of food and your colon is empty of fecal waste so you can eliminate the dead yeast from your body as fast as possible before you feel foggy and achy from the die-off. So if feel you need to do a candida cleanse because you have candidiasis, the fungal infection caused by an overgrowth of yeast, I recommend doing it today.

It's easy to do and only takes a few minutes to execute. Add two tablespoons of birch xylitol to a glass of warm water. Drink it down along with your other drinks and then stay close to a toilet a few hours later for the die-off effect. The yeast eats the xylitol granules made from birch bark (looks just like white sugar) but cannot digest it. *Definitely* do your coffee enema on a day you do a xylitol flush.

FOLLOWING YOUR GUT

Gut feelings tell you what to take in, what to reject and what to spit out. They tell you when to relax, when to go grazing, and when to go on the hunt. It's gut instinct that tells you to do something on impulse, like cross the street just in time to bump into an old friend — or avoid an accident. Gut feelings give you a sinking feeling in the pit of your stomach or butterflies of excitement. They tell you what you really hunger for in your life in the largest sense possible and in each moment of a split-second decision. The effect of gut instinct is instantaneous and also long-lasting.

Gut feelings *are* the bodymind connection. They express at the visceral core of our embodied consciousness. When you get a gut feeling, you might feel it all over your whole body. The gutbrain has its own neurology and way of sensing, knowing and communicating with your nervous system. Via the vagus nerve, your hypothalamus receives chemical messages from nerve cells in your cranial brain and coordinates them with messages it's receiving from nerve cells in from your gutbrain. That crosstalk regulates a host of functions that sustain our bodymind health, including our inflammatory immune response to infection or toxicity as well as neurohormonal responses to changes in our environment or situation.

A gut feeling is a deep knowing in our emotional bodymind that is intimately connected to our feelings of hunger and attraction (I'm hungry for this, I want this, I'm going for it) or disgust, revulsion and aversion (this smells/tastes/feels rotten, I'm out of here). Physically, gut feelings tell you what, when and how much to eat and drink. But if your digestion is healthy, your gut is free of chronic inflammation, and your colon is unconstipated, gut feelings can tell you so much more.

Gut feelings can whisper an insight quietly in your ear like a refrain until you "hear" it and become consciously aware of it. Or they can scream in your face once in a blue moon in response to a highly unusual situation you've never been in before, like when you're literally lost in the wilderness, disoriented and about to panic and make a fatal error. Gut feelings can also express as a preference in your life that takes years to fully manifest. For example, gut instinct told me to retire early from university teaching before the shooting spree crisis in schools became almost a weekly occurrence. *"Are you sure you want to leave education after you've been a professor all these years?"* my mother asked. *"Yes Mom, I'm sure, it's a gut feeling."*

Ignoring your gut feelings can be a source of regret and illness later because you can only ignore gut feelings for so long before they express somatically as symptoms. The gut is very expressive this way because of the thinness of the mucosal membrane between our gut and the rest of our body, but also because of the connection between gut instincts and the limbic, emotional brain through the vagus nerve, that super-freeway for brain-body communication that runs along our spine and connects our visceral body to our brain. The crosstalk going on via the vagus nerve coordinates our digestive system, endocrine system, nervous system and immune system. Bottom line: if your gut is unhappy, you will be an unhappy person. And if your gut is unwell, you will be an unwell person. Because your gut is connected to the rest of you.

Let's face it, it can feel liberating and exciting to follow your gut intuition but it can also feel scary because gut feelings are impulsive and beyond the reach of your mind's cognitive manager. Gut feelings are different from rational thoughts and often challenge them. They often defy reason. That's why we say *"listen to your gut"* to someone who has a tough decision to make or someone over-thinking a choice to the point that they convince themselves to ignore their gut feelings and choose less than what they really want. Because it's your gut that's going to tell you if you feel satisfied at the end of your life, and whether you found what you had really hungered for. It will be a gut feeling.

Body metaphors

Body metaphors for gut feelings are visceral. *"It takes guts to do something like that,"* we say about someone who took a risk and beat the odds, or who performed an act of bravery under duress, or pursued a vision no one else saw. Or we say *"gut instinct kicked in"* to explain a sudden last-minute change that saved the day. When we decide to skip an ordeal by not engaging, we say, *"I didn't have the stomach for that."* When an event is painful and traumatic, we say it was *"gut wrenching"* and *"hard to swallow."* About a negative, stressful situation, we say *"it made me sick to my stomach."* If the stressful situation is long-lasting, we say *"it ate away at me."* To describe the impact of an insult or betrayal, we say it felt like a *"punch in the stomach"* or a *"kick in the gut."* About relationships, we might say a relationship *"turned sour"* or felt *"poisonous."* Or positively, we might say *"I had a good feeling in my gut"* about a person we just met. Or we feel butterflies of excitement about a new project or idea — or when we fall in love. And we say *"follow your gut"* to someone who is confused, because when you don't know what to do, everyone knows to *trust your gut.*

It takes guts to trust your intuition

If you are a person who is used to living in your head more than your body, changing your relationship to your gut intuition can be challenging. It's frustrating when someone asks you how you feel and you tell them what you're thinking, and then they say, "Yes, but how do you *feel*?" It's frustrating when you realize you don't really know how you feel because you don't really *feel*. And the reason is because you're running through life motivated by stress in flight-or-fight mode bypassing your gut feelings and trying to manage them with your smart mind while suppressing emotions that nonetheless surge up at the most inopportune moments to start a conversation that you don't want to have because it seems irrational. Or better yet, supra-rational — beyond reason and deeply emotional. Guttural even.

Honestly, gut feelings can be messy. But life is messy sometimes, isn't it? Especially if you're carrying around a lot of waste in your life from all the things you thought you wanted that didn't satisfy you. Following your gut takes courage. Help yourself out by cleansing your gut, feeding it and taking care of its waste so you can better sense, hear and embody your gut instinct to be well and to be happy in life.

Guts over fear

In a culture that has exalted the cognitive rational mind, giving yourself permission to follow your gut instinct, to be intuitive, or even to be *an intuitive*, can take an act of courage. For example, it takes guts to take your health into your own hands these days when the medical industry uses fear to sell the belief that we need pharmaceutical products every day of our lives to be well. It's gut instinct that tells you when you watch a pharma ad whether to trust the visual track showing happy actors seemingly enjoying a medicated life or to trust the scrolling caption in small print along the bottom of the screen speeding through a list of serious adverse effects of the medication being marketed. Imagine if the ad showed the reverse: a visual track of actors acting out every serious adverse effect of the drug being marketed and a tiny scrolling message at the bottom proclaiming the pharmaceutical drug will make you happier and healthier. Would you believe the ad? Would you buy the product? What does your gut instinct tell you?

When you check in with your gut intuition, it helps if your gut is uncongested, emptied of waste, hydrated and populated with beneficial bacteria. Because if your gut is constipated with fecal waste, dehydrated and populated with sugar-loving yeast, you may only hear OCD tics, anxiety and depression in the crosstalk between your gut and brain. Feeling disconnected from healthy gut intuition can leave you feeling overwhelmed, foggy and confused, and therefore susceptible to marketing messaging from the advertising industry telling you what to do in a time of uncertainty.

For example, gut instinct told me to decline the rushed-to-market Covid vaccines. I have many friends who took the Covid vaccines and the booster shots who still got Covid and got sicker than I did, who today are still afraid of catching a cold. Whereas I hardly think of a cold as a concern. Some of these friends now have anxiety over possible long-term adverse effects from the vaccines. And others who consented are now saying they wish they hadn't. They feel regret. One person I know experienced an adverse effect that was diagnosed as a vaccine injury by a medical doctor. Sadly, he consented to take the vaccine even though he was at low risk for severe or life-threatening symptoms because of his young age and good health. Now he has chronic pain and his life has changed — but not in the way he had hoped for when he took the vaccine thinking it would help him find work as an actor during the pandemic.

Take the time to check in with your gut when you make potentially life-changing decisions. Do you feel stressed or unstressed? Safe or threatened? Satisfied within and self-sustaining or looking for something external to consume? Your gut feelings are on when you are parasympathetic dominant (unstressed and calm) rather than sympathetic dominant (stressed and fearful). To hear your gut feelings, it helps to step out of the fear for a minute to reset before you make a decision. Gut feelings can be measured in your blood pressure, body temperature, inflammatory immune response, heart rate, respiration rate, moods, sexual arousal, appetite and thirst. If you blush red and catch yourself holding your breath with your heart pounding in anticipation with butterflies in your belly, that's your gut feelings talking. Listen in.

Taking care of chronic depression, anxiety, ADD and OCD

When you accept the gutbrain connection for what it is, you understand why thinking you can fix depression by popping an antidepressant in your mouth without cleansing, nourishing and restoring your gut is a fantasy of instant gratification that can end up making you more sick over time. Because that's a very disembodied way of approaching the problem of chronic bad moods. Whether it's depression, anxiety, ADD, ADHD or OCD, if you seriously want to take responsibility to make yourself feel better, you need to get real about the state of your gut health and the role it plays in modulating healthy moods.

Until you clear an overgrowth of sugar-loving yeast from your intestines for example — starve it of sugar and purge it — you may find it difficult to hear your gut intuition and gut instinct and feel happy about it. Instead, you may just feel a lot of disturbance in the field. Like a kind of depressive agitation accompanied by sugar and carb cravings, not to mention bloated, gassy belly, stomach aches and constipation. The same is true for cleaning out a dirty, constipated liver. Our liver acts as our body's glucose reservoir, releasing energy as needed into our bloodstream and keeping our blood sugar levels constant and stable. If you suffer from sugar highs and lows, or you've been warned about diabetes, take action now to cleanse and nurture your liver so it can function better.

Gut feelings of regret

Regret can come up when you feel your gut feelings in the middle of a fast. Starting with regret over all the crap you ate if you've been eating crap, or regret over what you've drunk and the things you've said or done. Things that went a certain way toward darkness and despair when they could have gone to the light happy place you feel sometimes when you're feeling in the mood. We all want that happy mood that's in the flow and free of all the bitterness and bitter tears.

Taking a break from eating is so relieving if you've been overeating. And so many of us have. It's what Americans are notorious for. Eating too much. Consuming everything plus. We like our servings jumbo size. We invented the 24-hour supermarket so we could eat throughout our days and nights. Snacking. It would be funny if the consequences weren't so serious. The truth is, we could all live better without all that dehydration, constipation and gravity. All that weight.

What would we consume if we all stopped eating all that stuff that doesn't really nourish us? What would we consume in a consumer society to keep the economy going?

The answer is obvious. We'd consume everything that's good for us because it feels good in our embodiment. Meaning we can eat it and it leaves us feeling well instead of chronically sick. We'd invest in sustainable wellbeing and consume that. We'd follow our gut over fear-mongering advertising. Our gut tells us what is good for us and what is poisonous. Yes, you have eyes to see and ears to hear, but what does your gut tell you? Lay your hand on your gut. Is it happy? Is it sad? Is it hot and inflamed, or cool and feeling in the mood? Trust your gut. Listen to your gut feelings.

Below are a few exercises to help you tune into your gut intuition by helping you reset your vagal tone from stressed to relaxed.

GUT FEELINGS EXERCISES

Exercise 1: Vagal toning

If you're stressed out, vagal toning works fast to turn the stress down a notch so you can feel, sense and hear your gut intuition. Vagal toning can be used to switch channels from your fight-or-flight sympathetic nervous system (with its injections of cortisol and adrenaline running around putting out fires) to your parasympathetic nervous system with its steady flood of feel-good hormones, starting with serotonin and all her best friends — dopamine, oxytocin, pitocin and endorphins.

There are many vagal toning exercises. One of the easiest is to hum a primordial sound or seed mantra out loud. You'll feel the vibration throughout your body, and of course people around you will feel it too. I give you two well-known seed mantras below. And then we'll talk about how they work. The difference between these two primal seed sounds is that one is sounded with the lips closed and the other with the lips open. Try both and see which one resonates with you.

Om (\Ōṃ\). The primal sound of absolute consciousness in Hindu and Tibetan Buddhism.

Hu (\Hü\). The first word of creation in ancient Egyptian.

Sounding a primordial seed vibration in your vocal cords resonates a harmonizing vibration traveling both up from your throat into your brain and down through your heart to your gut through the vagus nerve. You'll feel it throughout your body — vibrating through your vagal nervous system all way down through your heart and through your gut to the bottom of your diaphragm. The sound will travel up as well into your hypothalamus, pineal and pituitary glands, into your cranial bones, and quite distinctly in the paper-thin sphenoid bone in the middle of your skull behind your eyes and above your palate.

As you repeat the mantra out loud, you'll notice your heart rate slows, your breathing relaxes, your blood pressure drops, your mind clears, your hunger fades and indigestion eases. You'll feel your moods elevate. If you repeat a sound mantra long enough, your mind will drift off at some point. It could be seconds or minutes. You may not know how long it was because when you "drop down," you drop into the timeless space of resting state connectivity. What you become aware of in this state is the bodymind connection where you hear the voices and sounds of your gut intuition.

To practice with these seed sounds, sit cross-legged on the floor and make yourself comfortable. Or sit in a comfortable chair. Inhale fully through your nose. Exhale the mantra out loud in your throat as you exhale your breath steadily to its very end. As you exhale the sound of the seed mantra, you will feel your abdominal muscles and diaphragm contracting slowly. At the end of the breath, fall into emptiness and hold for a count of 3. Then inhale through your nose from the bottom of your diaphragm and exhale the primordial seed sound again. Repeat the seed mantra 3-5 times.

Exercise 2: Belly down

Lie down flat on your belly on the floor on a carpet or yoga mat with your arms stretched out over your head with your palms, forehead, belly and tops of your feet pressing down into the floor. Gravity will compress your visceral organs (lungs, heart, organs of digestion, excretion and reproduction) and 3rd eye point (sphenoid bone, hypothalamus, pineal gland, pituitary gland). Practice silent nasal breathing on a 4-count inhale and a 4-count exhale. Tune into your interoceptive sensations of what is happening internally as you compress the organs and glands of the gutbrain connection.

Inhale fully through your nose and on an exhale through your nose press your left leg into the floor while lifting your right leg up off the floor a few inches. Hold the pose through a slow steady exhale through your nose and at the bottom of the breath slowly release your leg down to the floor. Inhale again fully, and on the exhale lift the opposite leg. Go back and forth lifting one leg at a time for 5 repetitions. This exercise is a fast way to compress your visceral organs and 3rd eye point while stimulating your vagal nervous system and awakening your gutbrain connection.

If you're agitated, stressed or angry and want to calm yourself down and shift the vibe fast, this exercise provides immediate relief. Pragmatically, if you're lying flat on the floor on your belly practicing silent nasal breathing and lifting one leg up and down and then the other, it means you're not walking around in circles agitated and adrenalated and causing all kinds of ruckus in the lives of the people around you. Children take this somatic posture instinctively when they feel overwhelmed. They throw themselves on the floor on their belly and kick their legs up and down. After a few minutes, they feel relaxed and calm again. Sometimes we would do well to copy them.

For the rest of your fast, rather than walk or storm around in the feeling of anger, agitation and overwhelm, use this exercise when that feeling gets triggered before you engage a fight or start one.

The somatic-emotional energy needs somewhere to release other than through your angry mouth and legs. Whatever is going on in your life, lie down on the floor immediately and start this exercise. It may look funny to people in your life, but they will intuitively understand why you're doing it and leave you be while you calm yourself down and gather your parts.

Exercise 3: Gut twister

Twisting exercises wake up your gut intuition because they fire up the gutbrain connection from your perineum to your pineal gland using a spiral twisting motion to simultaneously stretch your spine and vagus nerve and compress your visceral organs. Twisting poses also provide a reality check on the state of your gut.

The most common reason twisting poses can be challenging is because your gut is bloated, distended, inflamed, and full of fecal waste such that your belly is in the way when you try to twist. Visceral organs that are chronically stressed may feel hardened, inflamed and enlarged. If this is you, your lower back might hurt too because of the nagging strain from carrying so much weight, inflammation and waste in your gut. Accept the state of your belly for what it is. Work with it.

Sit on the floor cross-legged with your spine upright, crown of your head pointing up to the sky, casting your gaze into the horizon. Tuck your right leg in front of you and wrap your left leg on the outside of your right leg. If you feel challenged to sit on the floor cross-legged, then put your right leg out straight on the floor and bend your left knee to place your left foot outside your right knee with your left knee pointing up to the sky. Place your hands on the floor for support.

Breathe in through your nose. On the exhale through your nose, gently twist to the right in a gentle upright spiral placing your right hand behind your sacrum on the floor and your left arm on the outside of your right knee for support. While contracting your diaphragm, pull up your perineum (pelvic floor between your gonads and anus.) As you twist and contract your pelvic and abdominal muscles, you will sense your liver, intestines and colon compress. Twist as far as you feel comfortable without strain. Hold the twist for a 3-count at the bottom of the breath, contracting the muscles in your abdomen to accentuate the compression.

As you inhale, release the twist, gently returning to your centerline with your eyes gazing straight ahead of you into the horizon. Relax and take a breath. When you're ready, inhale and then on the exhale twist to the right again. Repeat 5 times. Then switch sides, tucking your left leg in front of you and wrapping your right leg in front of your left if you're sitting cross-legged. Or stretch your left leg out straight on the floor and bend your right knee to place your right foot next to you left knee. Breathe in through your nose and on the exhale twist to the left, placing your left hand on the floor behind your sacrum to provide support. Repeat 5 times. Keep your spine upright, avoid slouching. Give your visceral organs some room to breathe.

After you complete 5 repetitions twisting to each side, sit comfortably with both your hands cradling your belly. Ask this part of you what it would say if it had words. Then listen empathetically with your hands, ears and heart to your gut feelings.

DAY 7 FACE TO FACE

Chapter 10

FACE TO FACE —
Session Seven

Day 7 of the fast

One week of fasting is a milestone. You may be tempted to come out of the fast on Day 7 having reaped plenty of benefits. It's typical to have already lost 5 to 7 lbs. of weight from fat burn and from purging fecal food waste from your colon. However, after a week, fasting has gotten easier. The daily routine is old hat, and some deep metabolic, emotional and psychological healing is about to take place from now until Day 10. So stay in your fast if you're motivated to make these deeper changes happen faster.

Esther Perel, a popular relationship therapist who teaches relational intelligence in her books and games for couples, says that more than anything else, our relationships define the quality of our lives. I think all of us intuitively understand the truth of that statement. To live well and to feel happy, content and whole, we need healthy relationships with those around us. The changes taking place within you that you instigated by fasting will inevitably change how you relate to people in your life, because when you change, your relationships change. So today is a good time to turn your attention to emotional-relational issues you may be challenged by that may be blocking your sense of wellbeing. The lesson and exercises in today's session nudge you to do some work on how you relate to, communicate with and negotiate conflict with people in your life who care for you and for whom you care.

EMOTIONAL HONESTY IN RELATION

When someone in your life says, "I need to talk to you face-to-face," check-in with how your body is responding. Do you feel curiosity and happy to connect? Or do you feel dread, defensiveness and a desire for separation? Do you feel yourself settling into your emotional bodymind to listen with empathy and an open mind? Or do you find yourself putting on the robes of the judge, preparing your defense, and getting ready to take control of the situation? Maybe you feel yourself turning your back on the person and heading for the nearest exit door. Take note of your habitual, knee-jerk response and own it. Emotionally honest face-to-face communication starts first and foremost with being honest with yourself.

It's natural to do Fast Therapy with an intimate partner or with family members and friends, because it's easier to team up to run the kitchen and keep the drinks flowing. Sometimes while interacting with people in your life, conflicts may come up, people may bump into each other so to speak. When fasting in a group it's easier to hold a safe space to explore what's going on at a deeper level and get to the bottom of it. If you are fasting solo, it's a good idea to let people around you know that you're fasting and that you may at times detox blocked emotions that can affect relationship dynamics.

As your bodymind cleanses its waste, it becomes easier to express feelings and needs in face-to-face conversation with people. For people who are conflict avoidant, Day 7 is an opportune time to practice emotional honesty and the skill of conflict negotiation. As acidic waste is pushed from your visceral organs after a week of fasting, and your organs and endocrine glands become cleansed and nutrient-saturated, messenger hormones will be on the move. As a result, emotions and moods can flux with the tides. If you find yourself feeling icky, toxic and irritable today, help yourself out as well as the people around you who might find you irritating. Drink more fluids, take a binder like activated charcoal, walk to get some fresh air, and do your coffee enema, or even a second coffee enema, to help eliminate toxic waste faster. The emptier your colon is, the less irritated your bladder and the cleaner your liver, the easier it is to feel and express your authentic emotions.

Body metaphors

Body metaphors for emotionally honest communication when it matters most — including in public or in intimate conversation or during conflicts of interest — all refer to what you're doing with your face. *"Say it to my face!"* we say to someone caught talking behind our back. *"Look me in the eyes"* we say to someone we sense is lying to us or hiding their true intentions or emotions, or to someone who is turning a back on us. *"Look at me,"* we say to reassure people hiding their face in shame or embarrassment who need to feel respected. Or we say *"look at yourself"* when someone is wallowing in a mess that they created, or we say *"take a look in the mirror"* to prompt self-reflection. When people do something they later regret that created consequences they must now deal with, we tell them to *"face the music."* Or we say *"look the truth in the face"* to people who have been in denial. *"Face the facts"* or *"face up to it"* are common verbal prompts to get us to be more emotionally honest with ourselves about a situation staring us in the face that we've been avoiding. These body metaphors all guide us to be more emotionally honest when we communicate. They urge us to let our face come into alignment with our true feelings and intentions so that people around us can trust us and understand us and empathize with us.

When needs clash: negotiating conflict

If you find yourself triggered by someone or triggering someone, or both, you have a choice. Rather than walk away, block the person, or dig in and argue, what would happen if you looked that person in the face and made a conscious effort to connect? For those who are reactive and quickly triggered, give yourself a precious minute to take a deep breath and slow down. Tune in so you can listen better, starting with listening to your own heartbeat. Is your heart racing or calm? If racing, start by resetting your vagal tone from stress to rest-and-connect by bringing your awareness to silent nasal breathing on a 4-count inhale and a 4-count exhale. Maintain healthy boundaries by following some simple steps to enable safer conversations. They're easy to do if you practice them, and they work because they include authentic emotions and needs into the conversation quickly. The method is from the late Marshall Rosenberg in his classic book *Non-Violent Communication.* Non-violent communication can be done quickly and effectively in four easy steps.

Step 1. Make an observation of what happened without any evaluation or judgment.

For example, you might say, *"I just saw you roll your eyes when I said I was going to fast for 10 days,"* or *"I just heard you say 'I doubt you can do that.'"* Whatever happened, reflect exactly what the person said and/or did without evaluating or judging it. Just make a neutral observation of what happened.

Step 2. Say how you felt.

Search for feeling words. For example, you might say *"when I heard you say x, y, z, I felt uncomfortable, disappointed, sad, brokenhearted, helpless, embarrassed, or angry."* Whatever the feeling is, name it and own it. Be emotionally honest.

Not sure how you're feeling? Check in with your felt senses for body metaphors that describe what you're feeling in your body. Trust that our bodies tell the truth. For example, if someone says to you, *"when I heard you say X, my heart dropped,"* take that at face value. Avoid saying *"you made me feel x, y, z."* That's heading off in the wrong direction toward co-dependency and blame. Own your feelings. Nobody makes us feel what we feel. You'll notice there's nothing to argue about when you own your feelings. If I say I'm feeling sad, for example, that's how I'm feeling. No one can say, *"Oh Camilla, you're not feeling sad!"* I'm the only one who knows how I'm feeling!

Step 3. State what you need.

State your need in the most general way. For example, you can say, *"I need support to do this fast, lose weight, lower my blood pressure, clean up my diet, or detach from drugs or alcohol."* Or you might say, *"I need to talk with emotional honesty about our relationship,"* or *"I need more reciprocity in my relationship with you,"* or *"I need to start dating again after my spouse died."* Whatever it is that you need, say it out loud and own it the same way you own your own emotions.

Avoid saying *"I need you to...x, y, z."* Saying that we need someone to do something for us to get a need met is a set-up for disappointment. It's similar to saying someone made you feel a certain way — it's a sign of co-dependency and messy boundaries. The truth is, you don't need anyone to do something they can't do or aren't willing to do, just as no one can make you feel a certain way if you're feeling something different. You do have needs and you do **need** to get those needs met, and you do **need** clarity about whether the other person can meet those needs or not when there's a conflict of interest. That's what negotiation is all about. However, you may find it easier to get your need met somewhere else or with someone else. That's the reality.

Step 4. Make a specific request to get your need met in a way that gets a clear *YES* or *NO* answer from the other person.

You need to know where you stand. After making a neutral observation of what happened to cause the conflict, after saying how you honestly feel in your embodiment, after stating what you need, the final step in healthy conflict negotiation is to ask for something tangible that would help you navigate the current situation to get your needs met. Grammatically, the ask is a positive statement of what you need, preceded by a conditional question. Say something that sounds like *"Would you be willing to...x, y, z?"* For example, you might ask *"would you be willing to refrain from rolling your eyes when I'm talking?"* After you ask your question, stop talking and wait for the answer. Many people lack the skills to negotiate, and unless they ask you for help, you're wasting your time trying to teach them. Right now, all you need is a clear YES or NO answer to your request. Trust the body language if it differs from the words. If a person says, *"Of course!"* and then you see their eyes roll, take it at face value. That's a *NO*.

There is an art to negotiation, and some people are gifted at it whereas others who grew up in families that negotiated very little and argued a lot may be really challenged. Whatever your skill level, practice makes perfect. As you improve your negotiation skills, you quickly notice that it's easier to negotiate conflict successfully when you make a request that is good for both parties, that is for the higher good of everyone involved, and that liberates everyone because it shifts the conversation from arguing, coercing and manipulating to figuring out how to get everyone's needs met in good faith. It's called a win-win and it's the golden key to healthy communication.

Let's review. When a conflict arises, first make a neutral observation of what happened, then say how you felt when it happened, then state your need, and then ask for something specific that would help you get your need met. Practice this method of non-violent communication with discipline, and you will liberate yourself and everyone else from controlling, manipulative and coercive communication that is less than emotionally honest. I can assure you that if people in your life are capable and want to give you what you need, asking with non-violent communication increases the likelihood that they will give you what you are asking for — especially if what you are asking for is for the higher good of both parties. If the person can't give you what you need, you need to know that so you can look elsewhere to get your needs met.

Let me give you a common example. Many people turn to a spouse for support when they fall ill. That's natural, and it's also healthy. It's far better to be honest about your mental, emotional and physical needs and ask your spouse for help getting those needs met than to hide the fact that you're ill to "protect" or "not worry" or try to "please" your spouse. It's better to be honest than pretend that you're not ill when you are. However, often a spouse doesn't know how to help. They just honestly don't know how. The best the spouse can do is to be honest and say they don't know how to help, and then assist in finding someone who does know. Maybe that means searching online to find an expert to help. Or maybe it involves reaching out to family and friends who might know someone who could help. None of this would happen if the person struggling didn't ask to get their needs met in the first place, even if the first person asked had to say NO. The asking and the answering get the ball rolling.

The same goes for getting your needs met when dating. We all know people who waste precious time in their lives dating people who are never going to be able to help them get their authentic needs met in relationship, when all around them are people who are available who easily could. It's best to say what your authentic feelings, needs and wants are at the beginning and be willing to take the answer at face value.

It takes courage to be up front about your needs and desires because you may have to face your worst fear. But facing your fear is better than being chased by your fear at every crossroad going forward. Be honest, say what you need, and then listen with empathy to what the other person needs. Between those two needs is where the true art of negotiation begins. Propose a win-win that liberates both people, and you'll win every time.

FACE-TO-FACE EXERCISES

Exercise 1: Eye gazing with a partner

Find a partner to eye gaze with. If you have an intimate partner, ask that person if they are available. Or ask a friend or family member. Sit comfortably in a cross-legged position facing each other. Use pillows or bolsters to make sure you're comfortable because you will be in this position for a while, and you want to be able to focus your attention on the eyes of your partner without distraction. If you can't sit comfortably in a cross-legged position on the floor, sit in chairs.

Practice silent nasal breathing for a minute or two with a 4-count inhale and 4-count exhale as you establish eye contact and drop into a meditative state. Give yourself some time to settle in. It may take a minute for both partners to let go of feeling self-conscious and release their habitual public face. All of us have one of these public faces, and we can use it to protect ourselves by keeping people at a bit of a distance. Eye gaze long enough to feel yourself let go of that public face.

Once you've locked into a mutual gaze, allow the focus of your eyes to soften. You can look directly into your partner's two eyes, or you can look at their 3rd eye point on their forehead. Or you can soften your gaze to see the light of the energetic aura surrounding your partner.

In this silent state with your *"eyes wide open"* allow yourself to "see" the body story of your partner with compassionate kindness and accept it for what it is. Though your partner is being silent, you can listen to the vibration of the body story that is sitting right there in front of you, facing you in a moment of quiet vulnerability. Everything that ever happened and the feeling of what happened is stored in body memories that have made each of you who you are in the present moment. Accept that the eyes are the windows of the soul and allow yourself to connect and communicate silently without words. Witness, see and feel. And let yourself be witnessed and let yourself be seen.

Continue eye gazing for about 5 minutes or so. When it's time, find a way to mutually bring the session to a close without words.

After your eye gazing session comes to an end, take a walk together and talk to share insights and feelings. Or sit and have a cup of tea together. How did it feel to see your partner like that? How did it feel to be seen like that? Were you more comfortable seeing than being seen? Or were you more comfortable being seen than seeing? What feelings came up for you? Where did you feel those emotions in your body? What did you learn about yourself? What did you learn about the other person?

Exercise 2: Negotiating a conflict that needs to be cleared

Think of a person in your life you have an unresolved conflict with. If you are free of unresolved conflicts in your life, you're finished for Day 7. See you tomorrow in "Heartfelt" for session 8. However, if you have an unresolved conflict with someone that matters to you, fill out the chart below with three one-sentence statements and one clear question. Keep it short and sweet and to the point. Be emotionally honest. One sentence each. After you complete the chart, memorize the sentences and put the chart away to reference later.

When we negotiate needs with people in our lives, we are using multiple self-care skills. I hope these all sound familiar to you — eliminating negativity in your speech and finding peace in your words, listening with empathetic ears and activating your observing Self, being in touch with your emotions and diving beneath the surface to listen to your gut instinct, as well as saying what you need in good faith in a way people can easily understand.

Statement of your observation of the event/conflict:

_____

_____

Statement of how you felt when it happened:

_____

_____

Statement of your need:

_____

_____

Question that asks for something tangible and actionable to get your need met:

_____

_____

Next ask the person you have a conflict with to do this partner exercise with you in person or on Facetime or Zoom. Face-to-face is better, but you can also talk by voice on the phone. If the person is unavailable, or they decline your invitation, or they have passed away, then find a partner to stand in their place and role play.

Sit comfortably and face your partner. Start with your observation and work through all 4 steps of non-violent conflict negotiation, saying what happened, how you felt, what you need, and making your ask for a win-win that liberates everyone.

Go into the exercise free of any expectations, and you will be pleasantly surprised by the revelations that emerge about your own patterns of communication when it comes to negotiating your needs and other people's needs in relationship. Observe what is easy for you and notice what is hard for you. Be aware of where you are challenged. Some people are naturally caretakers who find it easy to hear the needs of those around them but who struggle to say what they need. Others know very well what THEY need and feel blindsided to realize that others have needs too. Some people who have been traumatized have a hard time feeling their feelings and are challenged to say how they felt. Leave your judgements outside the door of this exercise. Just take note of where you are personally challenged. Everyone is different.

When you do this exercise, bring your awareness to what are you feeling in your body. What are you sensing? Where in your body do you feel those feelings and sense those sensations? What happens for you when you say what you feel or what you need? What happens for you when you hear the feelings and needs of the other person? What happens for you when someone says they can't or won't help you get your need met? What happens for you when someone gives you what you need with ease because you've asked in a way that is easy for them to understand and empathize with, and because they get their needs met too? Track any changes that you feel in your body.

Keep in mind that social science studies show that the skill of negotiating conflict with language is in place by age 5. If your family didn't teach you this skill, cut yourself some slack. When you're 5 years old, it's clearly not your fault! Even if everything goes awry on your first try at this exercise, trust that the way to acquire a skill is to practice it.

DAY **8** HEARTFELT

Chapter 11

HEARTFELT —
Session Eight

Day 8 of the fast

By Day 8 of a 10-day nutritional wet fast, you've lightened the burden on your heart because you've given your liver and kidneys time to cleanse and restore your blood. Both of these organs filter your blood of waste, pathogens and toxic substances, and play a role in regulating your blood pressure. Your liver also plays a role in regulating blood cholesterol and stabilizing blood sugar. Clean, healthy oxygenated blood takes stress off your strong but vulnerable beating heart — that core organ at the very heart of everything, pumping your life's blood day in and out and keeping the pulse of your conscious embodiment. Make sure you walk today and breathe in fresh air to fill the wings of your heart with oxygen.

The lesson and exercises in this session nudge you to do some deep emotional healing of your heartfelt feelings. Take heart in knowing that healing heartfelt emotions happens faster when your blood is cleansed, hydrated and oxygenated, and when waste has been filtered from your blood and eliminated through your liver/colon and kidneys/bladder. Today is an optimal time to take care of unresolved matters of the heart that may have been weighing you down in the past and causing heartache.

EXPRESSING FEELINGS OF THE HEART

A heartfelt hug, thank you, apology or condolence feels authentic and sincere because it comes from the heart without pretense. Heartfelt feelings express love, desire and attachment as the impulse to hold what's dear to you close to your heart. They give you courage when what you love is threatened and motivation when you have mountains to climb and oceans to cross to reach a beloved person or goal. Heartfelt feelings express as a sense of deep longing, telling you to reach for what you really want and to trust your heart's desire, even if you feel incredibly vulnerable doing so.

Ignoring heartfelt feelings, covering them up, or trying to hide them or suppress them can make you sick at heart. Being heartsick for too long can make you sick all over, because our heart is connected to all the rest of us via the vast reaches of our cardiovascular system. The heartbody connection is why holistic practitioners say *"a heartfelt feeling that cannot find its expression in tears will cause other organs to weep."* Heartfelt emotions like grief, sadness and despair, or love and joy, can express through our eyes as emotional tears loaded with prolactin and oxytocin — bonding hormones that enable us to connect with each other in times of need. For this reason, it's healthier to let a cry out than to stifle it. Vice versa, rarely crying or being unable to cry at all can be a sign of hormone imbalance, damage to mirror neurons, and blocked communication between the heart and brain.

The vagus nerve that runs along your spine and connects your gut to your brain also connects your heart to your brain. Neuroscientists today know that Descartes got it wrong when he thought *"I think, therefore, I am."* The heart sends more messages to our brain than our brain sends to our heart. It's our heart that is the center of our consciousness. And to a great extent that Enlightenment way of thinking that our mind is separate from our body has caused so much of our postmodern condition of chronic ill health and separation from each other and our environment. Thinking *"I feel, therefore, I am"* is a healthier way to live a fully embodied life.

The vagus nerve and its branches create a superhighway for crosstalking neurotransmitter hormones that determine whether your heart beats fast with stress hormones (adrenaline and cortisol) or beats slow and calm with feel-good hormones (serotonin, prolactin, oxytocin, dopamine and endorphins). Your vagal tone affects not only your physical heart health but also your emotional heart health, your moods including empathy, compassion and connectedness, your mental health including your ability to focus and to think clearly and logically, as well as your somatic memory including remembering who you are, where you are, and where your keys are — especially the keys to everything that really matters to you and your loved ones. Healthy crosstalk among your heart, brain and body orchestrates your ability to act in the world and to respond to people in your life in meaningful ways that maintain heartfelt social connections.

Body metaphors

Body metaphors for heartfelt feelings and their effects in our lives have to do with making a heart connection or losing that connection. We say, *"his heart wasn't in it"* about someone who left his job, career, marriage or labor of love after a false start or a long struggle. Today, we *"heart"* something we love in social media. And we describe the central innermost part of something as its heart, as in *"the heart of the story."*

Sometimes heart metaphors have to do with the location of heartfelt sensations in our body. We might say *"I felt my heart in my throat"* when we go to speak and a wave of raw emotion swells up to the point that our voice shakes or we feel speechless. Or we might say *"my heart sank"* when we feel disappointed.

When we describe an act of kindness that takes courage or sacrifice, we say a person has a *"big heart."* And to *"take heart"* means to gather your courage and lift your spirits. When we *"take something to heart,"* it means we not only understand something but also accept it emotionally. And when we say we *"learned something by heart"* it means we understood it deeply and committed it to body memory. When a person is *"open-hearted,"* it means that person is capable of giving and receiving love and compassion. Likewise, when we say to a person, *"come on, have a heart,"* we are asking for compassion and kindness.

The heart's field of metaphors is so vast because the reach of the cardiovascular system is so vast. The tempo of heartfelt emotions can vary widely, like your heartbeat, in response to social situations. They can be lightning fast and spontaneous, as in *"my heart sank at the sight of him"* or *"my heart jumped for joy at the sight of him."* Or they can feel deeply rooted and long-lasting, like my friend's heartfelt desire to prevent teen suicide after her son committed suicide.

When we say, *"follow your heart,"* we mean follow your heart's desire. Hold in your arms what you hold dear in your heart. Seek connection with what you love and who you love. Nurture those connections, care for them, protect them. Since home is where the heart is for most of us, following your heart means going home in some way. And I'll say even for those for whom home is where you hang your hat, the first and last home we all have in this lifetime is our body. Our embodiment. Coming home means to come back over and over again to the heartfelt feelings that tell you who you are, what you need and what you want, and what your purpose is in this lifetime.

Your body knows the truth of what is, and what could be, because you have the heart for it. Your body knows what you want and who you love and what you're going do about it. Follow the heartbeat of your happiness. Reach out to touch someone you care for.

While your smart mind will play a role in the *how* of it, divine consciousness will ultimately be in charge of the details if you allow your heartfelt feelings to set your intention and direction. And so we say, *"trust your heart"* and *"don't overthink it!"* That means surrender to being led by your heartfelt feelings rather than by your head and thoughts, follow the emotions pulsing within you. Go home to your heartbeat when it is calm, content and connected. When it is flowing with love and compassion and empathy. Imagine living your life like that, open-hearted and connected.

Anyone who has held a person in their arms while they died knows the power of a heart-to-heart connection. The same is true for newborns. Just being in the same room when a person is born does it. It's a heartfelt bond for life that expresses the deep structure of our mammalian nature to form lasting social connections. To love and to be loved through thick and thin, in illness and in health, until death do us part.

Visceral needs of the heart

Heart disease is the number one cause of death in the U.S. Isn't it time for all of us to take better care of our hearts? Our hearts have visceral needs for healthy foods including healthy fats, amino acid proteins, and minerals and vitamins from plant foods that are high in nutrients and low in toxic substances. Our hearts don't need processed foods with sugar and transfats; they need real whole foods. Our hearts also need enough clean water to hydrate and prevent dehydration. And we all need the right balance of electrolyte minerals for healthy fluid exchange to prevent both edema and dehydration that stress our heart. We also all have a need for a healthy gut that excretes waste after every meal, and a healthy liver to filter our blood, and healthy kidneys to regulate our blood pressure and fluid levels, because all these functions together prevent chronic stress on our heart.

When we do our own personal healing work, healing heartache is really a priority. Our heart has emotional needs that, if left unmet for too long, feed systemic bodymind illness and unhappiness because of the heartbrain connection and the heartbody connection. Take responsibility for getting these needs met, beginning with admitting to yourself and the people in your life that you have them. Today, rather than suppress these needs, let yourself feel any heartache you are carrying within you. Touch it and listen. Start an emotionally honest conversation with someone in your life who is connected to your heartache and speak from your heart rather than from your head. You'll find the conversation goes much better.

Choose feeling words to stay connected to your heartfelt feelings. Speech acts that get heartfelt needs met are healing and empowering, whereas thoughts and speech that habitually block you from getting your heartfelt needs met can become maladaptive and cause more illness and heartache over time. Avoid overthinking! Trust your feelings. It takes courage sometimes to express honest heartfelt emotions that have been blocked and suppressed, but there's a reason we say it feels good to *"get it off your chest."* Because if you don't, it becomes a heavy weight on your heart that you carry with you everywhere you go. So get it off your chest today. And be willing to hold space for the people you love to do the same.

Keep in mind that people who suffer chronic liver stress and inflammation may vent a lot of anger when they express their feelings, but that's a stressed-out liver taking over the crosstalk between mind and body. Until the liver cleanses its waste, it's hard to hear the heart talk. Some people who have chronic kidney stress may vent a lot of fear when they emote, but that's their stressed-out kidneys taking over the crosstalk. Until the kidneys cleanse their waste so they can better filter the blood and regulate fluid levels and blood pressure, it's hard to feel the heart's faith and courage. Why get angry about that? Accept the bodymind connection for what it is.

However, once your liver, kidneys and gut cleanse and restore, your heart feels more peaceful, calm and less stressed, because healthy kidneys and healthy adrenal glands that sit on top of them downregulate stress hormones. In the same way a healthy gut upregulates feel-good hormones that shift you from fight or flight to rest and connect. Because you've taken care of yourself by fasting, you can reach out today and connect with love and empathy more easily. It's what we all need more of these days. Be proud of yourself for taking the time to cleanse your liver, kidneys and gut in order to care for your beating heart so you can connect with people in your life in heartfelt ways.

Living a heartfelt life

When you *"trust your heart"* at a critical choice-point in your life, or when making a difficult decision that will change your trajectory, you are accepting the role that heartfelt feelings play in guiding you to the happiness, love and contentment we all naturally desire. Our hearts feel most at peace when we feel connected to our authentic core self and to others for whom we care and who care for us. The sooner we accept that need for what it is, the sooner we can honor it as a daily practice.

We all need more heartfelt emotions in our lives. Only heartfelt feelings will get us from where we are at the end of the Age of Reason with its chronic postmodern condition of bodymind illness into a new Age of Empathy that feels healthier and more sustainable and that is more about creating lasting peace than fighting wars that never seem to end. Think of it as a future present in which humans embrace the intelligence of the heart again and honor it for what it is. Everything that matters. Everything to hold dear. Everything to love.

HEARTFELT EXERCISES

Exercise 1: Reaching for your heart's desire

Lie down on the floor on your left side with your knees bent. Place a pillow or rolled up towel under your head for support so that your neck is comfortable. Stretch your arms straight out in front of your chest, with the palm of your right hand resting on the palm of your left hand. Close your eyes and visualize what you really want right now in your life. Imagine your heart's desire as if it has already happened.

When you visualize what you really want for yourself, imagine the sensory details. What do you hear when you put yourself in the middle of your ideal manifestation one or two years from now? What do you see when you look around the scene? What do you smell? What do you feel on your skin? What do you feel in your heart?

When you complete your visualization of your heart's desire, open your eyes, take a deep breath in and as you slowly exhale reach out with your right hand for what you want with your whole heart. Slowly slide your right palm over your left palm and beyond it across the floor as far as you can reach. Sync the reaching motion with your slow deep exhale. The reach will activate your shoulder and ribcage to get involved and all the visceral organs that are attached with fascia to your ribs. Your hand will pull your arm and shoulder into the reach and also will pull your spine into it, and your head will make adjustments to roll with your torso. Explore how far you can stretch out your right arm as you reach as far as you can for what you want. Put your heart into it. At the bottom of the exhale with your arm fully extended and your hand reaching out as far as it can go, hold the emptiness for a 3 count.

On an inhale that starts deep in your diaphragm inside your visceral core, slowly draw your outreached arm back to its original position until your palms are touching again. Then keep going, sliding your right shoulder back until your shoulder is pointing behind you, your chest and heart open to the sky, and your top arm bent at the elbow resting on your ribcage.

Repeat this reaching out and retracting in cycle of movements 5 times with your right arm, and then switch sides and reach with your left arm. As you practice reaching, visualize what you really want deep in your heart. Notice if the left side feels the same as the right side. Maybe one arm can reach farther than the other. Notice the differences.

Exercise 2: Heartfelt forgiveness

In order to take care of our heart, we all need to come to peace with whatever happened in the past, accept the situation now in the present moment, and forgive people in our lives for the things they did that hurt us. In the same way, we need to forgive ourselves for choices we made that hurt others, including people we love and care for but also strangers we didn't know. The people who hurt you don't need to know you are forgiving them. Likewise, those you hurt don't need to know you are forgiving yourself for what you did in the past. Honestly, it doesn't matter if they are dead or alive. It doesn't matter when the hurt happened. All that matters is that right now, in the present moment, you open your heart to forgiveness. Do it for your own heart health.

Name of a person you hurt.   **Name of the feeling of the hurt.**

_____   _____

_____   _____

(Ex: Betrayal, abandonment, disrespect, etc.)

Statement of self-forgiveness:

I open my heart and forgive myself in this present moment for hurting _____.

Name of a person who hurt you.   **Name of the feeling of the hurt.**

_____   _____

_____   _____

Statement of forgiveness:

I open my heart and forgive _____ in this present moment for hurting me in the past.

Exercise 3: Making a heart-to-heart connection — partner exercise

Stand facing your partner and make eye contact. Reach out with your left arm and place your left palm on your partner's chest close to the heart. Respect privacy if your partner is a woman and place your palm on the chest above the breast. Have your partner mirror you, reaching out with their left hand and placing it on your chest close to your heart. Both partners place your right hand on top of your partner's left hand resting on your chest. This creates a circuit of energy moving in a circle between both partners' heart chakras.

Take a deep breath in and let it out slowly while maintaining eye contact. Practice silent nasal breathing in and out, softening your gaze until you can see the energy field around your partner while you feel their heart through your listening hand. Take in your partner's presence without judgment. Look into their eyes to see their soul. Listen to your own heartbeat pulsing beneath your partner's touch. Is your heartbeat fast, anxious and stressed? Or is it slow, calm and relaxed? Listen to the heartfelt feelings pulsing there beneath the surface of your ribcage.

Then shift your attention from your own heart to your partner's. Tune into what you're sensing through your listening left hand resting on your partner's chest close to their heart. Listen with empathetic touch to the heart-talk of your partner, and to the feelings of the heart, while looking into your partner's eyes. Connect in this heartfelt way without words.

Be an empathetic witness if someone cries heartfelt tears during this exercise. Stay present and experience what's happening in your sensory body and in your heart and heartfelt feelings when you connect with someone who is crying. If it is you who is crying, allow yourself to feel the emotions in the tears and to be seen in your vulnerability by your partner.

When the time feels right to both partners, find a way to silently disconnect your hands from each other and bring the exercise to an end with a heartfelt hug.

DAY 9 SCAR TISSUE

Chapter 12

SCAR TISSUE —
Session Nine

Day 9 of the fast

By Day 9 of nutritional wet fasting, your body has entered a state of accelerated autophagy, or self-consumption. It is a state of self-cleansing in which our immune system's macrophages degrade and recycle (phagocytize) whatever is non-essential within us that is weighing us down and draining the energy of life, including parasites (worms, fungus, pathogenic bacteria and viruses), tumor cells and toxic carcinogenic substances from the environment, as well as damaged, dead and dying cells. We all have experienced an accelerated state of autophagy when we've run a fever to fight off a viral or bacterial infection. When we survive the fever, a few days later, we feel great having lost a few pounds of body fat. Wasting away can be a good thing if you are infected with parasites, growing tumors, are poisoned and inflamed within your core visceral organs, or walking around with too much body fat and a high toxic bioburden. Sometimes, it's just time to take out the trash.

A fever is a way to do that fast. But why wait until you are sick to take out your trash?

During autophagy, lysosomes, our cellular garbage collectors, carry out bits and pieces of cellular waste into intracellular lymphatic fluid to eventually be purged from the body in sweat, mucus, urine and feces. Sometimes it comes out in tears. Today is a good day to walk and talk. Break a light sweat and instigate some deep breathing of fresh air with someone in touch who can be all ears, and who is available to be your partner for a trauma release exercise. Reach out and connect. Definitely do your coffee enema today to help yourself out. For those of you who are fasting for the first time, you're probably astounded at how much waste is still coming out of you after 9 days of fasting.

Autophagy also plays an essential role in wound healing. It is our embodied way of clearing away damaged and dying tissue around a wound and triggering the fascia to heal by stitching a fibrin scaffold in the wound site that healthy cells can attach to. Stitched into that fascial scar tissue that heals the wound is the emotional body memory of the wounding. That memory of wounding needs to heal too, needs to be integrated and stitched into our conscious embodiment in the present moment. Otherwise, the physical wounds heal but the psychological wounds don't. Sometimes, it's just time to heal the pain of the past and grow some new skin and connective tissue.

Because of the synergistic effect of autophagy and detachment, Day 9 of a 10-day fast is an optimal time to do some personal work around healing unresolved trauma from the past that you'd like to let go of today. Today is a good time to touch your wounds old or new to trigger some new growth. The lesson and exercises in this session nudge you to locate and release somatic-emotional body memories of past pain and injury that seem to come out of the blue with tremendous energy when triggered in the present.

HEALING TRAUMA

When you heal from a trauma, there's pain; expect it. But there's something beyond the pain of healing that comes with restoring functional use of that vulnerable part of yourself that was injured. Whatever way you were traumatized, the healing process is the same. Accept that you are wounded, injured or ill. Let go of pretending to yourself or to the people in your life that it is anything other than what it is. Own your traumas — the injuries and scars and the healing in between.

Scars are the physical embodiment of being injured as well as the perceptual, sensory and emotional memory of the experience. But scars are something more. Between the injury and the scar is the healing, and so our scars are a living testament to our power to heal.

Healing is a process that takes time. Give it time. Feelings will come up about what happened to you that injured and traumatized you and made you who you are today. When a healing crisis comes up, surrender to the pain and release of it. There may be irritation, loss, outrage, fear and regret to feel, process and release. But understand and accept in your heart that full healing happens when you stop compensating and start using that injured part of yourself, even if it means stressing scar tissue and growing yourself in new ways. Only by testing and challenging whatever function you have at each step of the way can you stretch and strengthen old wounds to regain more functional use of your whole Self.

Scarred for life

Everything about a scar is meant to last a lifetime. The fibrin stitching that mends a wound with scar tissue lasts the rest of our lives, as does the body memory of injury and pain. Bessel Van Der Kolk's bestselling book on trauma is entitled *The Body Keeps the Score* because the body remembers and never forgets. The book became an immediate bestseller, to date translated into 14 languages, because what van der Kolk describes in detail about post-traumatic stress (PTSD) from his clinical research as a psychiatrist is something we can all relate to.

The English word *"trauma"* comes from the Greek word *"traumata"* which means to pierce or to wound, and the Sanskrit word *"turah"* which means wounded or hurt. To be traumatized is to be injured, wounded and hurt. Our vulnerability to being wounded and scarred is part of our human condition. Any of us can be injured, traumatized, and scarred for life. When that happens, our mind can protect itself by suppressing the memory of pain, but our body remembers. For this reason, van der Kolk recognizes when working with post-traumatic stress that somatic approaches that engage the body directly are far more effective than talk therapy, cognitive behavioral therapy and psychiatric drugs in helping people heal.

It's important to recognize that trauma in one part of your body affects your whole bodymind because of the vast web of fascia that holds all our parts in relationship — nerves, glands, organs, bones, muscles and lymphatic structures are all interconnected in a web of fascia that has its own nervous system, much like your skin. So save yourself some time and avoid thinking it's just my knee, back, arm, spine, womb, breast, heart, head or teeth. Yes, it is that part of you where you were injured, but it's so much more. Trauma anywhere in your bodymind can affect the functional use of your whole Self — including physical, physiological, metabolic and reproductive abilities but also your ability to feel, express and regulate your emotions, think clearly and make sense of reality, and to connect, bond and communicate with people in your life about the things that really matter to you. And they matter to you because you live with the scar tissue and body memories of them.

Body metaphors

As a noun, a scar is the physical mark left after your body repairs and heals a wound, and so scars can be used as metaphors for both the memory of trauma and also the healing of trauma. Bestselling author R. H. Sin put it poetically: *"The pain means you're alive. The scars mean you've survived."* John Steinbeck wrote, *"To be alive at all is to have scars."* In these usages, scars are metaphors for resiliency in the face of life's challenges. Rose Fitzgerald Kennedy famously wrote after the assassination of her two sons John and Robert Kennedy: *"It has been said, 'time heals all wounds.' I do not agree. The wounds remain. In time, the mind, protecting its sanity, covers them with scar tissue and the pain lessens. But it is never gone."*

Just as a scar is a body metaphor for the trauma of being injured, injuries can be used as metaphors for feeling hurt and wounded. For this reason, people might say *"it cut me to the bone"* or it felt like *"a stab in the back"* or a *"punch in the stomach"* to describe psychological and emotional pain that wounded them. Some people who have chronic psychological and emotional scarring from longstanding abuse may cut their skin or subject themselves to self-sabotaging ordeals in order to externalize the woundedness they are feeling within and to trigger a physical healing crisis in which endogenous endorphins are released to relieve pain.

20-minute rule for somatic-emotional release

When a body memory of trauma gets triggered, the memory stored in that part of the body will discharge emotional energy from the original trauma. Hands-on practitioners call this somatic-emotional release. When working with somatic-emotional release, mind your timing. A release usually lasts about 20 minutes. It can start at the drop of a hat and seemingly come out of the blue, or you can see it coming for a long time on the horizon. But once it starts, it usually lasts about 20 minutes from beginning to end. It's called a "release" for a reason. The body memory releases a tremendous charge of emotional energy that connects to physical sensations and perceptions. Like a wave on the ocean, the energy rises up, crests and then resides.

Emotional energy releasing through the bodymind can cause flushing and heating of the face and skin or shivering cold, dilation of the pupils, increased heartbeat, deep or shallow breathing, crying, sighing, shaking, whimpering, sobbing in pain, holding of the breath, clenching of the jaw and fists, storming around, collapsing to the floor, curling up small or extending the body as big as possible, freezing and dissociating, pacing around like a trapped animal, or acting like a child. Somatic-emotional releases can get very intense. And then, as quickly as they began, the somatic-emotional energy releases and dissipates. It's common afterward to laugh out loud and feel totally relaxed.

For Fast Therapy, we want to facilitate this natural process of somatic-emotional release rather than block it in any way. If strong emotions make you uncomfortable, remember the time frame. In the span of a lifetime, 20 minutes is a brief flash of time in which to witness and listen empathetically to a somatic-emotional release for someone you care for — or to experience one yourself. In our modern society, we are conditioned to suppress these "primitive" feelings. Give it the time. In *Brainspotting*, David Grand describes holding space for a somatic-emotional release of a trauma memory as riding in the vortex behind a comet. Stay in the tail of the comet, he advises, riding along in the acoustic, vibrational energy wave of it, and follow the comet wherever it goes.

Recognizing post-traumatic stress

People who have been traumatized may express symptoms of post-traumatic stress metaphorically in their speech. It's very important that we recognize these expressions when we hear them. They are doorways to the body memory of a traumatic experience that you might easily miss. Develop an ear for these body metaphors of PTSD, because the sooner you recognize them for what they are, the faster you can respond in a way that is healing rather than re-traumatizing —

whether the person expressing post-traumatic stress is someone you are caring for, or is you.

For example, you might hear someone you care for suddenly say *"I feel empty inside"* or *"I feel invisible"* to describe a state of victimization, powerlessness, loss of strength, splitting of self, or loss of control over self and life situations **(dissociation)**. Or someone might respond to an event in the present as if they were experiencing a past traumatic injury again, saying things like *"I thought I was being attacked"* when they weren't **(re-experiencing)**. Or someone might be drawn by an *"inexplicable attraction"* or *"compulsion"* to repeat something potentially injurious again, sometimes even flirting with catastrophe that looks self-destructive or self-sabotaging **(reenactment)**. Likewise, a person might feel a protective impulse to *"step back"* or *"step away"* or withdraw like *"a turtle into its shell"* to circumvent situations that might trigger a trauma memory **(avoidance)**, all the while grieving over or complaining about the lack of meaningful social contact or intimacy.

If someone you care for describes *"a mood of worry washing over me"* or a *"wave of anxiousness"* seemingly rising up out of nowhere, be aware that a memory of trauma might have been triggered that stimulates the brainbody to turn up the adrenaline and cortisol in anticipation of looming danger **(anxiety)**. When we hear someone we care for express an aversion to social situations that can't be controlled, it helps to understand that a traumatized, wounded part of that person may be expressing a lack of trust in self and others that can lead to illogical thinking and socially awkward behavior **(impairment in cognitive and social skills)**. Keep your ear out for *"I can't stand"* or *"I hate"* statements and behaviors that limit the person's ability to function in the world, such as *"I hate conflict, crowds, driving, going to the dentist, public speaking, dating, intimacy, messy emotions, crying, etc."*

When scar tissue gets triggered

At times during the healing process, scar tissue will get triggered. Count on it. Once triggered, body memories of trauma discharge emotional energy and sensations spurred by an associated somatic-emotional experience in the present that connects to the body memory of that traumatic ordeal in the past. The survival function of somatic-emotional discharge of traumatic body memories are obvious; if you ate from a plant that poisoned you once and you almost died, you want to remember the details of the experience so that you don't do it again. Peter Levine in his classic book on trauma *Waking the Tiger* uses being attacked by a tiger as a metaphor for the somatic experiencing of a traumatic ordeal. If you survive a tiger attack once, you certainly don't want to have to do it again. So while your family and friends are playing around the campfire, it's you who maintains hypervigilance enough to spot the tiger's head staring at you through the flickering shadows in the bush. That's a good thing, right? However, when a person who was traumatized by a tiger in the past spends every day for the rest of their life anxiously looking for tigers everywhere they aren't, it's time to do some healing work around the body memory of that trauma to release the charge and reset the nervous system from stress mode to rest and connect mode.

When the body memory of a traumatic experience is suppressed and the conscious mind is not aware of the cause, a person whose body memory of trauma is triggered can suddenly feel as if they are re-experiencing the trauma again when they're not. It is as if the person is transported back to a past time and place where a traumatic ordeal is unfolding. In the case of the modern trauma of invasive surgery under anesthesia, the conscious awareness of the ordeal is physically suppressed, although we know now that people can hear under anesthesia though they cannot move their body — a traumatizing experience in and of itself.

Invisible scar tissue

Some of the most challenging scars to heal are those that aren't visible because the scar tissue is in an area of the body that is easily covered by clothes such that only intimate partners or close family members would ever know about them. Some scarring can't be seen with the naked eye, such as an injury inside the brain or ulcerated tissue inside the gut. And fascial scarring can't be seen at all even on a CT scan or MRI — even though fascia is the largest organ in our body, comprises about 16% of our body weight, and holds about 25% of our body's water. Fascia is loaded with nerves just like our skin. It has its own nervous system and endocrinology and transmits messenger hormones between the body and the brain via the vagus nerve. Fascia is literally the bodymind connection, and it is the holder of traumatic memories that our mind may be unconscious of.

In cases where scars exist beneath the surface of the visible, it's easy to misperceive scar tissue and the body memory of trauma. We may misrecognize what is right in front of us, mistake it for something else, project our own needs and desires onto it, or suppress it and forget about it once we do become aware of it. Hold this wisdom close to heart when doing healing work with the embodied memory of trauma, whether processing your own memories or empathetically witnessing and holding space for someone you care for.

Hands-on practitioners are aware of invisible fascial scarring because they can feel it in their hands as tight knots, tension and restrictions whereas healthy fascia glides and slides; it doesn't stick, restrict and bundle. Clients who seek help from a practitioner have a sense of where fascial scarring is because of the pain it can cause. Sadly, many people with chronic pain from fascial scarring are told *"it's all in your head"* and are treated with psychiatric drugs or painkillers. Or they may be treated with cognitive behavior therapy and talk therapy that don't really address fascial scarring and the unconscious somatic memory of trauma stored in fascia. Treating trauma in these ways can actually cause more trauma, whereas somatic therapies work directly with the body and its memory of injury to get better and faster results.

People with traumatic wounds, injuries and scar tissue that we can't see need our attention and emotional support just as much as those who have visible scars. Think of veterans who come home after suffering concussions, often multiple concussions, who may look okay on the outside compared to vets who have visible scars and missing limbs, yet who are suffering from traumatic brain injuries. The same for women who have suffered sexual trauma, or a traumatic birth, or children who experienced chronic neglect or abuse early in life. Just because you don't see the psychic, emotional, mental and physical wound and its scar tissue doesn't mean it isn't there.

SCAR TISSUE EXERCISES

Exercise 1: Name the injury/trauma

This is a naming exercise to help you bring unconscious trauma memories into your consciousness where it is easier to talk about them and work with them therapeutically. You will create four simple sentences in which you name aspects of the traumatic injury that left its imprint on you.

First, write down a brief statement of your injury/trauma in one short sentence. Name whatever it was that hurt and wounded you. Next, name the part of you that was injured. Then name the emotion that went with the trauma. Finally, name what you lost in functional use of your whole Self because of the ordeal.

If you suffer chronic mental, physical and emotional pain but lack a clear cognitive memory of an injury, describe your pain, its location, and the emotions and loss of function that go with it.

Statement of traumatic injury and pain:

_____

_____

Part of you that was injured:

_____

_____

Emotion you felt at the time of the injury:

_____

_____

What you lost in function:

_____

_____

Exercise 2: Touching the body memory of trauma

Touching the fascial network around the part of you that was wounded is a fast way to access the body memory of that injury. Search for an area of restriction, blockage, discomfort or pain. For example, I can touch anywhere on my pelvic bowl to feel the stress lines from the trauma of pelvic surgery over 20 years ago. I don't have to touch the scars themselves to connect with that wounded and vulnerable part of myself because it affected my whole pelvis. For example, I can hold my pelvic girdle in my hands by touching both my hip joints with my fingers while my thumbs wrap around the iliac crest, or pelvic ridge, above each hip. That places my palms flat along the sides of both wings of my ilium bones. Those big bones attach in front with fascia forming the pubis, and in back with fascia to the sacrum and tailbone. Sometimes when my pelvis is out of alignment, one iliac crest will be higher than the other, and as a result my gait will be off. If I try to walk very far like that I can quickly get into a pain body. Better to take a few minutes to touch the problem directly in my body to help my pelvis come back to balance before I take off for my day. I can use the feedback from my hands to help over-compensating muscles and stressed fascia to relax, allowing my pelvic bones to come back into alignment.

Once you make contact with the part of you that was wounded and injured, listen to the body story held there. Get a feel for it. Be all ears. Open your eyes and your heart. Ask that injured part of you to tell its story of pain and discomfort. What do you feel in your listening hands? What do you hear in your listening heart? If this part of you could talk, what would it say? Have an emotionally honest conversation with that wounded vulnerable part of yourself. Ask that part of you what it needs to heal.

Exercise 3: Share your body story of injury with a partner

Person sharing: Ask someone who cares for you to spend 20 minutes with you to process your body memory of traumatic injury. The purpose is to share what happened and the feelings and sensations you experienced with an empathetic witness, in order to both discharge emotional energy from the body memory and to create a new memory to map onto the original one in which you feel resourced and supported in the present moment.

Sit on the floor or in chairs facing your partner. Start this exercise with a few minutes of eye gazing. When you are ready, bring the eye gazing to a close.

Using verbal language, intonation, and facial and bodily expressions, share your story of injury with your partner with whatever details stand out in your memory. Place a listening hand on the part of yourself that was wounded. While you recount what happened, let your eyes move anywhere they want, and let your body emote. Follow the feeling of what happened wherever it leads you.

When you get to the end of your story and you feel complete, check-in with yourself. How does it feel to be witnessed in your vulnerability? Did you feel comforted? Was it hard for you? Do you feel relieved?

Were you able to emote? Did you feel strong emotions rise up? Or did you feel you floated through the experience while observing yourself checking out? Share your experience of the exercise with your partner and discuss.

Partners: While the person you are witnessing for shares the body story of what happened and the feeling of it, place a listening hand on their shoulder or on the back of their heart. Make yourself comfortable so you can maintain empathetic listening touch as the story unfolds. With your words and intonation, reflect what you are hearing and seeing without interrupting the flow of the story. Focus on listening, witnessing and reflecting. When the story is complete, help the person integrate the past and the present by talking with them about their insights.

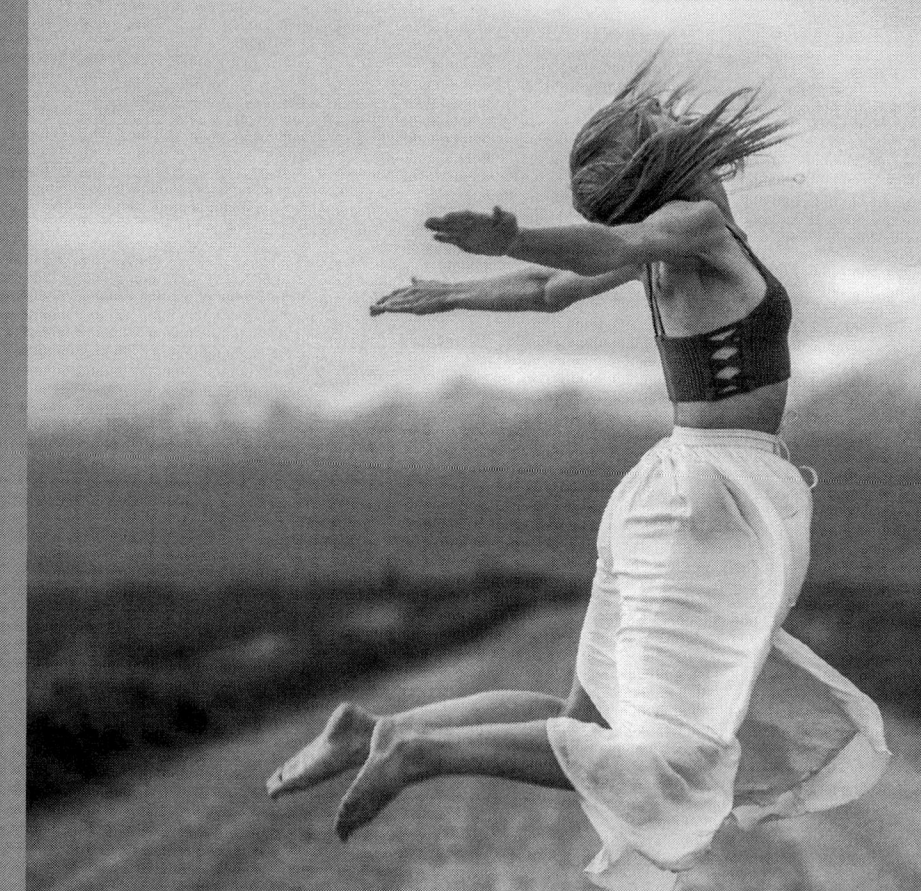

DAY 10 — LANDING ON YOUR FEET

Chapter 13

LANDING ON YOUR FEET — Session Ten

Day 10 of the fast

By Day 10 of fasting, it's typical to have shed 7-10 pounds of excess body fat and fecal waste, depending on how much body fat and waste you started with. Check the skin on the bottom of your feet and elbows, your tongue, and the whites of your eyes for visible signs of regeneration happening everywhere inside you — including visceral organs you can't see. With your intestines empty of excrement and inflammation quelled, the changes can look and feel dramatic.

Today is a good time for self-assessment and self-congratulation; enjoy the emptiness and detachment you've created within yourself by fasting. Rejoice in it, feel it, and walk around in it. Because tomorrow, it will be time to eat, chew and digest food again. And when you do that, your internal state of detached emptiness and heightened awareness will shift. So today is also a good time to integrate all your parts and visualize next steps. Because tomorrow you will have some choices to make. This session is intended to help you land on your feet after fasting so that those next steps you take are made in a state of balance and alignment. The exercises will help you get your feet under you and drive momentum for healthy changes after fasting.

GETTING GROUNDED

Our feet enable us to walk the Earth and are often referred to as humble servants for the load they bear on the journey of life. In old age, the day we can no longer stand up and walk is the day we have begun our final decline. To stand up vertically on two legs defines us as human beings and distinguishes us from our four-legged friends. However, while standing up on two feet gives us certain advantages, it also subjects us to an anatomical vulnerability. Losing our balance and falling down is a risk we all live with every day of our lives. We depend on our two feet to create stability, balance and shock absorption as we dance our way between the force of gravity weighing down upon us and the force of momentum pushing up from our feet when we stand up tall and step out into the world to take action.

What you do in the next 30 days after a 10-day fast sets a new bodymindset for healthier self-care, because it lands you at the proverbial 40 days to embody a new habit. In the divine synchrony of the bodymind connection, 40 days is also how long it takes a healthy liver to regenerate itself so that it can better filter your blood, the River of Life, and take stress off your beating heart. So do your last coffee enema today to give your liver some love and care. Of course, after today you can walk yourself right back into the old habits that made you want to fast in the first place. But after ten days of fasting, you've detached from your unconscious habits enough to have clarity about how little you really need to be fulfilled, happy and healthier.

Fasting teaches us the abundance of austerity, and the liberation from suffering that comes with living a more austere lifestyle by simply self-regulating our own consumption and waste. Fasting teaches us how little we all really need to consume, and nurtures within us the power of free will to live better by wanting less. And by standing up for what we do really need — clean drinking water, essential nutrients, less waste — with conviction and foresight.

In the past, many of us have lacked the emotional honesty to talk candidly about the ways in which we have made ourselves sick as individuals and as a society. And now, because we live in a time when so many of us are of chronically out of balance and falling ill, it's urgent that we each stand upright, look out into the horizon to see what's coming, and change course — starting with changing what and how much we consume and how much waste we have created from our attachments to things that are unhealthy for us. If you don't need it to be vital and well, skip the part where you pay for it. Don't buy it. Stand up on your own two feet and walk away.

Body metaphors

We all want our feet to carry us on our journey through life with grace, balance and stability, to carry us all the way home to safety and better health. And we want to be able to pivot in life and change directions to stay in the flow, and to be able to think on our feet and stand our ground. Our feet are part of our root chakra, connected by tracks of fascia to our legs, rectum, tailbone and immune system, and up through our spine to our head, jaws and eyes. If your jaws and eyes are out of alignment, you suffer chronic neck and back pain, and you feel foggy and out of balance, check your feet.

Body metaphors about our feet have to do with feeling grounded. Grounded implies we have our feet under us and feel balanced, in solid contact with the Earth. It means we can stand up on our own two feet and see what's in front of us (where we're going) and what's behind us (where we've been) and what's to the sides (the unexpected that comes from left field). It means we can move and adapt in the face of all kinds of obstacles and hardship that can trip us up and throw us off balance, putting our bodymind health and safety at risk.

The phrase *"landing on your feet"* evokes the feeling of a positive outcome after a period of trouble or difficulty. It suggests taking a fall and being able to get back up on your feet, or jumping over a precipice and landing upright in a balanced condition or state of being, or traversing challenging terrain without getting hurt. For these reasons, the phrase is often used to refer to recovery after illness, injury or trauma. When an obstacle trips you up and you land on your feet, it means you have come back to balance and arrived successfully at a good destination. All of us trip and at times fall on the journey of life. Whatever happened that gave you a tumble, focus on getting your feet under you before you hit the ground.

Feet symbolize your free will; your feet walk the path you choose and reflect how you choose to get there. If you want to avoid a certain path, turn around. You can drag your feet, stomp your feet and cry, get cold feet and let life step all over you. Or you could gather your parts for the journey ahead and get your feet under you before you head out with a clear sense of direction. Be willing to put your best foot forward after your fast, and you will have the world at your feet. Now that you've gotten your foot in the door of preventive self-care, take your next step forward in the right direction, keeping your eyes on the stars and your feet on the ground.

Set your compass to this quote about bodymind integration from Lance Secretan, a British author and inspirational speaker on inspired leadership: *"Authenticity is the alignment of head, mouth, heart and feet — thinking, saying, feeling and doing the same thing — consistently."* Add *"eating"* to his list to make this adage perfect for our purpose today. Choose consciously where you put your feet in relation to your mouth, head and heart after your fast is over. Make sure all your parts are in alignment, then walk the path to better health and happiness and stay the course.

An inspirational story about falling down and getting back up on my feet

I'll leave you with a personal story about landing on my feet after falling down in a dramatic downward spiral. It happened fast. Within the first few months of this painful ordeal, I went from being athletic and active to so unstable and unbalanced on my feet that I could barely walk up the stairs of my 3-floor condo without holding on to the handrail with both hands. At the worst stage of my healing crisis I was crawling up the stairs on my hands and feet. My knees swelled with fluid like balloons, and I had to have them drained with a syringe and needle seven times. My sacrum became stiff, inflexible and out of alignment with the bones in the back of my pelvis, causing me to feel ungrounded and to lose my natural gait. The physical and psychological pain was excruciating. I felt unable to coordinate simple movements as my joints entered a state of chronic inflammation. I went from doing chair pose in yoga to needing a toilet riser to get up and down off a toilet. Emotionally, I felt mortal fear and horrible anxiety, and depressed.

What happened?

The speed of my decline pointed to an environmental rather than genetic cause. During the pandemic, I rented a house for a month on a lake near my parents in Georgia because I wanted to be close by to help them if they got sick. They never got sick, but I was soon to find myself in need of help myself. Every day I would walk barefoot across a long, manicured lawn of perfect green grass numerous times to the dock to enjoy the stunning sunrise and sunset views, do my yoga practice, stretch my legs, play on the lakeshore and get fresh air.

However, the last week of my stay I noticed by knees were becoming red and inflamed, and I felt stiff doing yoga. I suddenly became more aware of my environment and noticed a detail I had missed before — *there were no weeds on the lawn.* Even along the shoreline where one would expect to find a variety of weeds where the water meets land, there were none. Turning detective, I opened a tool shed on the property. My heart sank. Two jumbo-sized bottles of RoundUp herbicide stared me in the face. I knew deep in my gut what the implications were because I've experienced a poisoning ordeal before when a dentist drilled a mercury amalgam dental filling without safety precautions to protect me from breathing mercury vapor. When you realize there is a toxic poison inside of you, it's a sickening feeling.

The active chemical in RoundUp is glyphosate, and I was aware it has been associated with non-Hodgkins lymphoma and gut dysbiosis (loss of beneficial bacteria) in class-action lawsuits. Was glyphosate also associated with joint inflammation? A quick search online confirmed my worst fears; I found the work of Dr. Stephanie Seneff connecting glyphosate to both osteoarthritis and rheumatoid arthritis. Glyphosate is similar in its chemical structure to the amino acid protein glycine that our body uses to metabolize and repair collagen and fascia. Glyphosate disrupts normal connective tissue repair and growth.

Diagnosis — osteoarthritis

In the month following my visit to Georgia, I fell into a state of chronic inflammation and irritation. The places in my body where I had scar tissue were the first to take a hit, starting with my knees (athletic injury) and pelvis (from surgery to remove an ovarian tumor.) I became disoriented and retreated to my bedroom where I wallowed in my pain. Eventually I was able to gather my parts to make an appointment with a knee surgeon who had easily removed a piece of torn cartilage in my knee a few years earlier. The orthopedist examined my swollen and inflamed knees, took X-rays, and diagnosed me with osteoarthritis. To my shock, my new knee X-ray when placed next to my X-ray from just a few years prior showed the cartilage in my knees had diminished by about one-third. In the weeks that followed, his two physician's assistants patiently drained my knees of fluid every week or two with a large needle and syringe before my crisis peaked and I began to recover. It was a harrowing and painful experience.

I now recognize people suffering with arthritis everywhere I go. I'm very aware what the symptoms look like and feel like. Over 53 million Americans suffer with this chronic degenerative condition to the point that many people think arthritis is just a normal part of aging. But happily, I'm here to tell you it's not. Three years after my ordeal, I live free of any symptoms of osteoarthritis.

Getting back on my feet

It took me a few months to gather my parts to do the 10-day nutritional wet fast, but I finally managed it. I felt better afterwards, but I knew I wasn't done. Three months after my first 10-day nutritional wet fast, I did a second one. I felt myself gaining momentum. A month after the second nutritional wet fast, I did a 3-day dry fast — no food and no water. In total, I lost 21 lbs. of damaged tissue and looked like skin and bones. But the inflammation was gone.

The most stinging memory from this challenging time in my life is the number of people in my community who said something to the effect of, *"It's just old age, Camilla, you'll get used to it."* I was blessed that my friend Anaswara, a yoga teacher, knew it wasn't "just old age" when I went within a few months from being an advanced practitioner in her classes to unable to do child's pose without using two blocks because my knees, sacrum and lower back were so inflamed, stiff and painful. She kindly offered me her backyard ice bath whenever I needed it — and so I ice plunged several times a week for a several months to take down the runaway inflammation. I started with 3 minutes of ice-bathing and worked my way up to 8 minutes, long enough to take down the inflammation and trigger a rush of feel-good hormones — endorphins (endogenous pain-relievers), serotonin (the happy hormone), and dopamine (the pleasure hormone that tells you to wake-up to your senses in the present moment). Plunging in an ice bath also helped me clear my head and stay focused.

Ice bathing and fasting share the same characteristic of putting your body in a controlled healing crisis to trigger an altered state in which healing can happen faster. In both practices, the goal is to get in fast and stay in long enough to feel the effects. Honestly, 3 to 8 minutes in an ice bath is a blink of an eye in the span of a lifetime. Just about anyone can do it. But so is 10 days of fasting from eating food. In both cases, if you think you can't do it, the blockage is psychological and mental, not physical.

As the inflammation and pain diminished and my head cleared, I got my bearings enough to reach out for help from the integrative physician in west Los Angeles who had helped me recover my health in the past after mercury poisoning from dental amalgam. Dr. Hans Gruenn listened to my story, said he had seen glyphosate poisoning before, and commented that it happens to dogs too. He held my hand, looked me in the eyes, and praised me for having the presence of mind and the discipline to fast to get the poison out. Then he recommended I take a teaspoon of glycine every morning and evening to help myself grow back healthy collagen and fascia. I left his office and ordered a half pound of glycine online for $19.99. What happened next felt miraculous.

Within weeks, I was growing healthy fascia again. I ate only organic whole foods that were herbicide and pesticide free, eliminated all inflammatory foods, and supplemented with a heaping teaspoon of glycine mixed in raw goat yogurt with a tablespoon of fish oil morning and night. Over the next nine months, I returned to my normal body weight of 135 lbs. and grew back healthy fascial connective tissue. Today I hustle up and down three flights of stairs between my kitchen and my office carrying a tray loaded with food and drinks, run around on the beach chasing the tide during golden hour, and power through sweaty ashtanga yoga classes. On my 65th birthday, I was back to throwing martial arts kicks for my Instagram feed.

It's healing for me to share my body story and to tell as many people as I can that you can heal from arthritis and other chronic inflammatory conditions if you move quickly. Arthritis is the number one cause of disability in the U.S. It's a painful and debilitating chronic degenerative condition that brings daily suffering and loss of function to tens of millions of Americans. What more do we need to know to take action to prevent arthritis by demanding a ban on glyphosate in the U.S. as many European countries have already done? It's up to all of us as consumers to step forward and take action to make healthy change. Refuse to eat this toxic substance on your food, drink it in your tap water if you live downstream from agricultural farms, or buy it and spray it on your lawn and garden.

If eliminating glyphosate from your internal and external environment sounds daunting to you, take heart in this inspirational message that came in the box my amazingly robust and fresh olive oil is shipped in from Flamingo Estate's owner Richard Christiansen. The package with its heartening message came just before Christmas. Given my experience with glyphosate, it was music to my ears.

> *"This holiday, we continue to give a percentage of all sales to Farmer's Footprint — and their efforts to ban glyphosate (RoundUp). It remains the most used poison in the world and has been detected in our water, breast milk, urine, clothing, and the food we all eat. It increases the risk of non-Hodgkin lymphoma by 41 percent, but has never been banned by the FDA. Farmer's Footprint is a coalition of farmers, educators, doctors, scientists, and business leaders working damn hard on our behalf. They are my holiday heroes, and I am so happy to continue giving money to them with every product we sell."*

If you need more than Richard Christiansen's inspiring words, try this quote from Abraham Lincoln: *"Be sure to put your feet in the right place, then stand firm."*

LANDING ON YOUR FEET EXERCISES

Exercise 1: Honor your feet by stretching them before you take off running

There are 26 bones and 33 joints in each foot, with over a hundred ligaments, tendons and muscles, all connected by fascia. Our feet are basically bundles of fascia that bind water, by which our feet act as shock absorbers to dissipate and disperse the impact of walking, running and landing on our feet after a leap or fall. We all need our feet to be hydrated but not swollen with edema. Foot baths with magnesium salts are a great way to detoxify and remineralize these humble servants that enable us to walk, run and leap through life with all its challenges.

Give your humble servants some love before you walk out of your house in the morning or at the end of a long day on your feet. Touch them, feel them and listen to what they need. Care for your feet so they don't become your Achilles' heel. Below are a few simple stretches to warm your feet up before you ask them to carry your load for the day or to soothe them after a long trek. It starts with sitting on the floor to touch your bare feet with your compassionate, listening hands. Warming up your feet will help you maintain proper balance and structural alignment throughout your body all the way up through your legs, pelvic bowl and spine to the top of your head, providing proper support for your eyes, jaws and teeth, neck and shoulders, and that sometimes aching back.

Sit on the floor with one leg stretched out and bend the opposite knee to place your ankle across your outstretched leg just above your knee so you can easily hold your foot in your hands. Do all the exercises with one foot before switching to the other foot.

1. **Stretch your ankle by flexing your foot up and down (dorsal plantar flexion).** Firmly grasp your lower calf above your ankle with one hand and hold the bottom of your forefoot in the other. Using your hands, gently but firmly flex your foot up

and down a few times to stretch all the fascial attachments to bones, muscles, ligaments and tendons.

2. **Stretch the subtalar joint by flexing your foot from side to side (supination & pronation).** The subtalar joint is below your ankle joint. Hold your heel in one hand and hold your forefoot in the other. Using your hands, flex your foot from side to side, stretching the outside edge until it extends down (eversion or supination) and then reversing and stretching the inside edge until it extends down (inversion or pronation).

3. **Stretch your transverse tarsal joint by twisting your forefoot to the left and to the right.** Grasp the bottom of your midfoot in one hand with your thumb grasping around your arch and hold the top of your forefoot in the other hand. Stabilize the bottom of your foot as you twist your forefoot back and forth, to the left and to the right.

4. **Stretch your toe joints by flexing and extending your toes.** Grasp the bottom middle of your foot with your thumb along your arch with one hand and hold your toes in the other hand. Extend your toes down as far as they will go comfortably, and then flex your toes up as far as they will go comfortably. If you've had toe injuries, be gentle and patient as you stretch scar tissue in your toes.

After you stretch one foot with all 4 warm-up exercises, stand up and balance on that foot. Notice your balance and stability when standing on that foot. Sit down and switch sides, doing all 4 exercises with the other foot. When you finish, stand up and balance on that foot. Compare balance and stability in both your feet.

Then, with both feet planted firmly on the ground shoulder width, ask your humble feet if they had words, what would they say? Listen with an open heart to your feet before you take your next steps.

Exercise 2: Visualize a future destination worth walking toward

For this exercise, sit comfortably with a journal or notebook close by. Close your eyes and practice silent nasal breathing for a couple minutes to drop down into a deep state of meditative relaxation.

Imagine yourself in a specific place a year or so in the future where you are doing something you love feeling healthy, happy and fulfilled. Envision it as a spacetime you can walk around in, rather than as a 2D Instagram selfie you look at. Put yourself inside the scene you are imagining. What do you hear as you move around? What do you see? What do you sense on your skin and in your gut? What do you feel in your head and in your heart and in your feet when you move through this space where you are completely content, feeling deeply fulfilled and well in your mind, emotions and body?

Approach your visualization as something that starts in your feet instead of your head. Ask yourself, where do you want to go in life? What is your ultimate destination? Where do your feet want to go when your head is spinning and your heart is hurting or you feel lost, stuck or ill? When you long for positive change about something in your life that's blocked and unwell? Something that needs healing that in your future visualization is already healed. Do your feet want to go home? Do they want to take a leap forward? Do they want to go back to find something that you lost along the way? Envision where you really want to end up and how you will feel when you have arrived at this optimal destination.

When you finish your visualization and feel satisfied, jot down in your notebook some details to remember it by. Then put your notebook somewhere where you know how to find it when you get lost or take a spill into ill health and unhappiness and need to remind yourself who you are and where you're going. Return to your visualization before you choose to run down the same old path repeating the same old pattern with the same disappointing result. Doing so will help you regain your footing after difficulty, get your bearings, and stay the course.

AFTERFAST

Congratulations. By diving into Fast Therapy and staying with the program for 10 days, you just embodied some fast changes. These changes will look different for everyone. For some they may be life-impacting, maybe even enormous changes at the last minute that turn your emotional, mental and physical health around. For others, they may be the first steps toward bigger changes coming. Either way, the changes you feel within you after fasting set you on the path to a sustainable wellbeing that you can feel. It gives you a taste of a life of less consumption and waste and more connection and feeling, and a sense of more optimal mindbody health. Good for you. So what happens next?

Coming out of your fast

Eating food after fasting is both a physiological and psychological experience. Consuming, chewing, and digesting food puts us in a different state of embodied consciousness from fasting, and it comes with different moods and feelings. Ideally, you want to make the transition between fasting and eating as gentle and easy as possible.

Just as there's a proper way to go into a fast to make it easier, there's a proper way to come out. For two days, eat only raw vegan organic whole foods — exactly the same way you went in. Raw food contains enzymes that help you digest and break the food down. Once heated, the enzymes are denatured, making cooked food harder to digest. Even if you came out of your fast before Day 10, you need two full days of raw vegan organic whole foods to transition with ease. Gently wake up your digestive system like you wake from a deep restorative nap. Sit down with a cup of hot tea first and plan your next steps mindfully. What's the rush?

There are two mistakes you want to avoid after a fast. Some first-time fasters may be chomping at the bit to eat a favorite cooked meal. I need to caution those of you fantasizing about eating a bowl of pasta or hamburger immediately after fasting that doing so will leave you sick to your stomach. The difficult to digest food will take a long time to drop down from your sleeping stomach into your duodenum and small intestine and will sit there decomposing. Decomposing is a kind word for rotting. It feels uncomfortable at the least, and at the worst, you'll be nauseous and constipated. I was foolish enough to try it once and I'll never do it again. A friend who is a gourmet vegetarian chef who was visiting took it upon herself to make me a delicious omelette with shitake and oyster mushrooms. Sounds harmless enough, and after declining for a few minutes I smelled the food and changed my mind. I wasn't listening to my gut intuition, and within fifteen minutes I felt sick to my stomach. Trust me, stick with modest amounts of raw vegan foods the first couple days after fasting.

Another mistake to avoid is forgetting to eat at all after 10 days of nutritional wet fasting. I know from personal experience it's easy to do. You find yourself in a state of being in which what you're going to eat today is absolutely the last thing on your mind. You may feel like you're flying high above any hunger at all and don't need anything external to feel content, awakened, energized and self-contained. That's a liberating feeling, but I caution you; fasting is different from starving yourself. If you stop drinking your daily drinks at the end of a 10-day nutritional wet fast and then don't eat any food at all, you are literally putting yourself at risk of falling down because you can become light-headed.

If after mastering this 10-day nutritional wet fast you can imagine yourself dry fasting (no food and no water), I get it. However, starting a dry fast after any kind of wet fast is the worst way to end a wet fast and the worst way to start a dry fast. It's a lose-lose either way. So please, follow the guidelines to stay grounded. If you're interested in dry fasting, I recommend reading Sergey Filonov's *20 Questions and Answers about Dry Fasting* to learn the proper way to dry fast. But one of the first things he says is never go into a dry fast immediately after a wet fast. He also says master a wet fast before trying a dry fast. So for now, focus on sourcing some organic whole vegan foods to transition out of your nutritional wet fast properly.

Walk through the organic produce section of your local grocery store or gather your parts to get yourself over to an organic whole foods market or a farmer's market. Touch the foods there and let them call out to you. Your gut intuition will tell you what you really need and want to put in your mouth. Let fast food be dead for you because it's dead food. Choose life. And avoid food packaged in plastic. Liberate yourself and the fish in the ocean swimming in plastic. Do it for yourself and for future generations. Take cloth shopping bags with you.

Pick out raw nuts and whole fresh vegetables and fruits to bring home to your kitchen. As long as the foods are fresh, unprocessed and herbicide, pesticide and fungicide-free they will be good for you. Ideally, you want to feed prebiotic and probiotic foods like sauerkraut to your beneficial gut bacteria before you consume cooked foods, especially if before your fast you craved sugar and flour and ran on caffeine with a shot of adrenaline. Feed your good bacteria and starve yeast in your gut to maintain the benefits of more stable moods and energy that fasting provides.

You'll be amazed at how much you enjoy eating whole raw foods and tasting their flavors and textures after 10 days of fasting. A single blueberry in your mouth after a fast can fill you with delight, as can simple carrot sticks dipped in raw hummus. Eating a salad of fresh lettuces, sprouts and herbs with chopped celery, red bell peppers, avocado and walnuts seasoned with olive oil and balsamic vinegar and sprinkled with bits of seaweed can feel like a meal fit for a king. Take the time to taste and smell the fresh whole foods you are consuming.

When you eat, bring your awareness to what you're doing in the present moment, because your relationship with the foods you consume is what really matters. It matters to you, and it matters to all of us together in a consumer society driven by consumer demand. Connect with your food. Savor each mouthful and chew each bite thoroughly. The slower you eat, the better after a fast because chewing aids digestion. Eat modest servings and leave time to digest and absorb your food thoroughly between meals. Hydrate to facilitate healthy digestion. Drink clean water an hour before and after eating but avoid drinking more than a few sips of water while eating because it dilutes your stomach acid. Always sit down to eat and take your time.

Returning to cooked foods

After two days eating raw vegan organic whole foods, the time has come to return to eating cooked food again. Make the transition graceful and gentle. Buy organic whole foods and cook your meals at home in your own kitchen. Take responsibility for your self-care after fasting. On the first day of cooked food after a fast, I like to start with spicy lemonade to assure I'm hydrated before eating, followed by a glass of kefir to feed healthy gut bacteria, and an hour later I eat a modest serving of hot buckwheat groats with raw butter or virgin coconut oil and a touch of maple syrup. I top it with a stone-fruit compote of apricots, peaches or plums simmered in a spoonful of raw butter. If stone fruit aren't in season, use fresh berries.

Please note the butter I use is raw. Once dairy products (milk, cream, butter, cheese) are pasteurized (heated at high temperature), the enzymes and nutrients in this superfood become denatured. Hence why pasteurized dairy is the most inflammatory food on the marketplace according to the FDA, whereas raw dairy is anti-inflammatory. If you can't find raw butter, use coconut oil instead.

For your main cooked meal of the day, I recommend a vegetarian stew that is hydrating and easy to digest. Every culture has recipes handed down for generations for hearty soups and stews that are nutrient dense and easy to prepare. If you need help in the kitchen cooking healthy foods, reach out to those in your family or community who know how to cook and ask for recipes. Ask for help but take your meals into your own hands.

One of my favorite post-fast dishes is *kitchari*, an Ayurvedic porridge used to restore gut health. The dish can be eaten for 3-10 days to cleanse and detoxify the intestines and colon. Kitchari is made by simmering basmati rice with soaked yellow split mung beans (moong dal), adding a root vegetable to the pot and toward the end adding a green leafy vegetable or two. The dish takes about 40 minutes to prepare and is considered a complete food.

The *chonk* (tempered ghee) that's stirred into a pot of kitchari at the end is made by gently heating a couple tablespoons of ghee seasoned with fresh spices like ginger, turmeric, cumin, fennel seeds, coriander, cardamom, and fenugreek along with a handful of cashews and golden raisins. It is served with a pinch of Himalayan pink salt (avoid cooking your salt) and a sprinkle of fresh parsley or cilantro with fresh ground black pepper. The dish is as delicious as it is healing. I assure you if *kitchari* is your first cooked lunch or dinner meal after a fast, you'll have a smooth transition. You'll also have a smooth bowel movement the next morning and feel great the next day.

Making your fast changes last

Because of the work you've done on yourself cleaning and restoring your internal environment, your true home, for just 10 days, you now have an opportunity to make the changes you've embodied by doing Fast Therapy last for a long time. Why stop now? Why go back to old habits?

All of us can adapt to the fast world we live in by managing our own consumption and waste and regulating our own emotional attachments to what is unhealthy for us. I invite you to become a self-regulating, self-sustaining human culturing a life of wellbeing every day of your life. Someone who cares. Someone who knows how to care — for yourself, for the people you love, and for the planet.

Remember this lodestar when you walk away from your fast into your new life of self-regulating consumption — if you wake up one day in the future feeling out of balance, sick at heart, in physical and psychic pain, and full of your own crap, you can always return to Fast Therapy for a fresh start on a newer, healthier, happier you. Invite a family member or friend to experience the power of self-healing through fasting therapy. When you set off on your journey, remember where you're going, and what it feels like to have already arrived.

ACKNOWLEDGEMENTS

I have deep gratitude for knowing my literary agent Bill Gladstone of Waterside Agency before he passed. He touched me and my writing with his vision to create and distribute books that bring knowledge, joy and wisdom to the world.

I am thankful to Samantha Skinazi for her stellar copyediting and her dogged focus on bringing the manuscript to completion. I needed those compassionate nudges.

This book has deep roots. One of them traces back to Dr. Gregory Ulmer at the University of Florida's Electronic Literacy Project for thinking critically that even our digital body has a mouth, and for his common sense understanding that the way to live well in consumer culture is to be strategic about what you put in it and how much. Sometimes, it's necessary to shut your mouth and stop eating it.

I was only able to believe that I could write anything lasting because of the early influence of Gail Shepherd in my life. She was, until the day she died, an amazing editor, poet and writer whose sensibility for words, and for the feelings beneath the words, touched so many people. I feel her voice guiding me from afar every time I sit down to write.

When Gail without warning stepped out of this world and I was left without my trusted reader, Sue Shepherd, her sister, stepped in to give the editorial feedback and support every writer needs to take a project from an idea to final manuscript. She has been a steadfast comfort and guide. Her sensibility as a fiction writer—she is the author of the novel *Animalia* and numerous short stories—helped me capture in words the healing body stories I share in this book.

Jenny Schmidt, a lifelong NPR writer and editor, helped me at a time of unbearable grief and loss to find my balance, see the bigger picture and stay on course writing and sharing stories that matter. For her influence on me from that moment on, I am eternally grateful.

Like most labors of love in life, there's family behind it. This book was blessed by three cousins. Natalie Boss—a colon hydrotherapist in Greenville, South Carolina—helped me deal with my own crap by showing me how to fast (shout-out to the staff at Pure on Main for the healing wisdom there.) Her influence on this book spans from conception to birth. Her sister, my cousin Gwynn Ross, has been looking over my shoulder with an encouraging gaze since childhood. Her heartfelt confidence kept me on path when writing was a struggle.

On the other side of my lineage across the Pacific Ocean, my cousin Alice Dixson, an actress in Manila, took fasting therapy to a new level by diving in to deal with a sleeping pill addiction and coming out on national live television to share this simple self-help remedy just about anyone can do—while warning viewers of the dangers of mixing sleeping pills with alcohol. Her emotional honesty inspired me to write a book that people in need could easily access.

Heartfelt thanks to long-time friends Alida de Paz and Cathy Dew for recognizing the thinker and writer in me, and for feeding my soul with good food and love of the creative act, not to mention helping me figure out how to simplify shopping lists, daily drink schedules and recipes.

My gratitude to Alexcia Panayotopoulos, shaman and poet, for journeying with me through Ayahuasca and San Pedro ceremonies to see the waking dream states of reality for what they truly are—universal stories as ancient as time of a human condition we all share. And for my yoga teacher, Anaswara, for exploring with me every possible holistic naturopathic pathway, including detoxification pathway, to greater health and wellbeing—while facing our family histories of chronic illnesses with courage, curiosity and an open heart and mind. I also thank Laura Fuller for a decade of intelligent and critical conversations about the future of body psychotherapy while walking the talk in LA.

I believe every teacher of writing should have to stop teaching after so many years and write their own book. It nurtures empathy in the classroom. How lucky I was to arrive at the English Department of

California State University at Channel Islands back in the day when Jacqueline Kilpatrick, Renny Christopher and Bob Mayberry had the common sense to institute holistic scoring of writing into the curriculum at the same time I was journeying into holistic health education. It helped me integrate the writer, educator and healer in me.

Last but certainly not least, I have immense gratitude for my wife, Marni Borek, for her help finding the way forward through the creative process while staying on brand. Because without a brand strategy these days, it's easy to get lost in the noise. She also fed the author in me with delicious organic homecooked meals that gave me sustenance and nurtured my heart, soul and mind from the book's start to finish. To say I respect and honor her support, creativity and guidance is an understatement of the deep, heartfelt feelings of my appreciation. This book came into its complete embodiment because of her.

Special thanks to photographers on Unsplash for photos that capture expressions of the emotional bodymind: Kunj Parekh, Kevin Fitzgerald, Priscilla Du Preez, Amir Esrafili, Toa Heftiba, Jakob Owens, Vadim Butenkov, Leonardo Zorzi, Motoki Tonn.

ABOUT THE AUTHOR

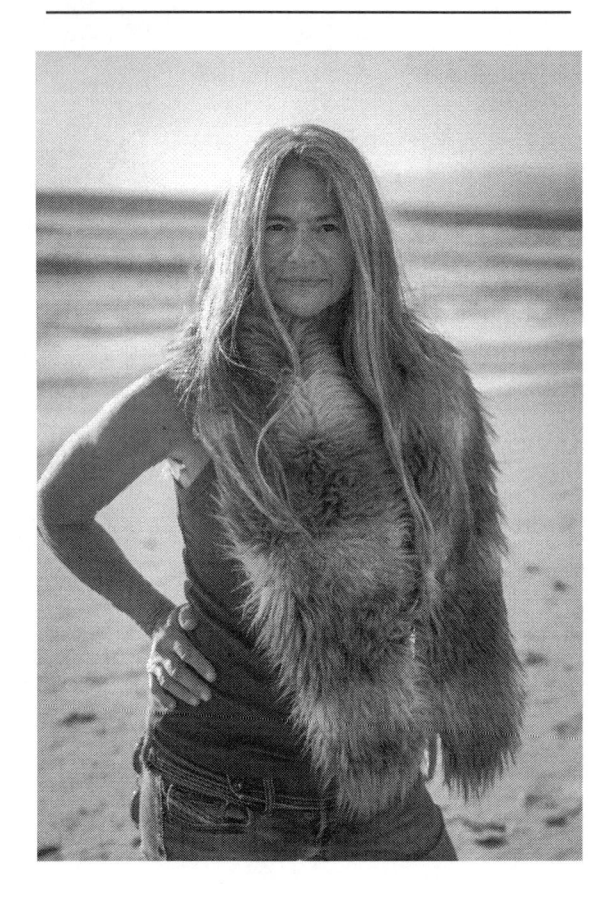

Camilla Griggers, PhD is a writer, holistic health consultant, and somatic therapist and educator in Los Angeles, California. She is the author of *Becoming-Woman*, co-director of the film *Memories of a Forgotten War*, and co-author with her mentor Ilana Rubenfeld of articles on somatic-emotional integration methods in *Somatics* and *The Handbook of Body Psychotherapy and Somatic Psychology*. A university professor for twenty years before pivoting into somatics, she brings a background in cultural semiotics and critical thinking to her training as a meditation instructor, holistic bodyworker and somatic psychologist. An educator at heart, she applies her broad knowledge base to educating the public about preventive self-care practices easily within reach that reduce the risk of chronic mindbody illness and support the development of lifelong wellbeing.

Made in the USA
Columbia, SC
06 July 2024